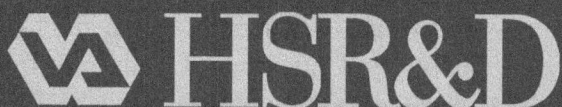

Teledermatology for Diagnosis and Management of Skin Conditions: A Systematic Review of the Evidence

January 2010

Prepared for:

Department of Veterans Affairs
Veterans Health Administration
Health Services Research &
Development Service
Washington, DC 20420

Prepared by:

VA Evidence Synthesis Program
Center for Chronic Disease
Outcomes Research
Minneapolis VA Medical Center
Minneapolis, MN

Principal Investigator:

Erin Warshaw, MD, MS

Research Associates

Nancy Greer, PhD
Yonatan Hillman, BA
Emily Hagel, MS
Roderick MacDonald, MS
Indulis Rutks, BS

ESP Program Director

Timothy J. Wilt, MD, MPH

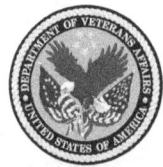

PREFACE

VA's Health Services Research and Development (HSR&D) Service works to improve the cost, quality, and outcomes of healthcare for our nation's veterans. Collaborating with VA leaders, managers, and policy makers, HSR&D focuses on important healthcare topics that are likely to have significant impact on quality improvement efforts. One significant collaborative effort is HSR&D's Evidence-based Synthesis Program (ESP). Through this program, HSR&D provides timely and accurate evidence syntheses on targeted healthcare topics. These products will be disseminated broadly throughout VA and will: inform VA clinical policy, develop clinical practice guidelines, set directions for future research to address gaps in knowledge, identify the evidence to support VA performance measures, and rationalize drug formulary decisions.

HSR&D provides funding for four ESP Centers. Each Center has an active and publicly acknowledged VA affiliation and also serves as an Evidence Based Practice Center (EPC) supported by the Agency for Healthcare Research and Quality (AHRQ). The Centers will each generate three evidence syntheses annually on clinical practice topics of key importance to VHA leadership and policymakers. A planning committee with representation from HSR&D, Patient Care Services (PCS), Quality Enhancement Research Initiative (QUERI), Office of Quality and Performance (OQP), and the VISN Clinical and Quality Management Officers, has been established to identify priority topics and key stakeholder concerns and to ensure the quality of final reports. Comments on this evidence report are welcome and can be sent to Nicole Floyd, ESP Coordinating Center Program Manager, at nicole.floyd@va.gov.

Recommended citation: Warshaw E, Greer N, Hillman Y, Hagel E, MacDonald R, Rutks I and Wilt TJ. Teledermatology for Diagnosis and Management of Skin Conditions: A Systematic Review of the Evidence. VA-ESP Project #09-009; 2009

TABLE OF CONTENTS

EXECUTIVE SUMMARY 1

    Background..1

    Methods 2

    Results 2

    Future Research Recommendations...7

    Conclusions..8

INTRODUCTION AND BACKGROUND 9

METHODS 11

    Topic Development, Technical Expert Panel...11

    Search Strategy 11

    Data Abstraction 12

    Quality Assessment...13

    Data Synthesis..14

    Peer Review 14

RESULTS 15

    Literature Flow 15

    KEY QUESTION #1 15

    KEY QUESTION #2 20

    KEY QUESTION #3 35

    KEY QUESTION #4 42

    KEY QUESTION #5 48

SUMMARY AND DISCUSSION...53

    Conclusions..53

    Future Research Recommendations...54

REFERENCES 56

TABLES

Table 1. Definitions of Outcomes 13

Table 2. Summary of Study Characteristics for Teledermatology Studies (KQ1, KQ2) 22

Table 3. Diagnostic Accuracy Using Histopathology/Lab Tests (KQ1a) 24

Table 4. Diagnostic Concordance -Teledermatology & Usual Care

    (In-Person Dermatology) (KQ1b)...27

Table 5. Management Accuracy Using Histopathology/Lab Tests (KQ2a)..................................32

Table 6. Management Concordance -Teledermatology & Usual Care

    (In-Person Dermatology) (KQ2b)...32

Table 7. Clinical Course Outcome (KQ3)..35

Table 8. Patient Satisfaction and Preference (KQ3) 37

Table 9. Time to Treatment/Dermatological Visits Avoided (KQ3) 41

Table 10. Cost Outcomes (KQ4)...44

Table 11. Key Elements for Success / Barriers to Implementation (KQ5)................................52

FIGURES

Figure 1. Reference Flow Chart...16

Figure 2. Quality of Store and Forward Teledermatology Studies 23

Figure 3. Quality of Live Interactive Teledermatology Studies 23

Figure 4a. Aggregated Diagnostic Accuracy: Store and Forward 26

Figure 4b. Primary Diagnostic Accuracy: Store and Forward...26

Figure 5a. Aggregated Diagnostic Concordance: Store and Forward 30

Figure 5b. Primary Diagnostic Concordance: Store and Forward 30

Figure 6a. Aggregated Diagnostic Concordance: Live Interactive...31

Figure 6b. Primary Diagnostic Accuracy Concordance: Live Interactive 31

Figure 7a. Management Concordance: Store and Forward 34

Figure 7b. Management Concordance: Live Interactive 34

APPENDIX A. Search Strategy..63

APPENDIX B. Data Extraction Form...64

APPENDIX C. Peer Review Comments and Responses 69

APPENDIX D. Abbreviations 72

APPENDIX E. Evidence Table: Overview of Studies for Questions 1 and 2.......................73

EXECUTIVE SUMMARY

BACKGROUND

Telemedicine uses telecommunication technology to transfer medical information. Due to the visual nature of a skin examination, telemedicine, specifically, teledermatology, may be a valuable tool in the diagnosis and management of dermatologic diseases for patients in rural areas (including rural Veterans Affairs Medical Centers and Community Based Outpatient Clinics) who may not have ready access to a dermatologist. Teledermatology may also be useful in primary care settings to triage cases and limit unnecessary dermatology clinic referrals. Although not the focus of this review, teledermatology may also be used to provide follow-up care or monitoring after an in-person dermatology visit. The objectives of this evidence synthesis project were to systematically review and summarize the scientific literature addressing: 1) teledermatology for the diagnosis of skin conditions, 2) teledermatology for the management of skin conditions, 3) clinical outcomes when teledermatology is used, 4) the cost of teledermatology compared with usual care (in-person dermatology), and 5) key elements of, and barriers to, successful teledermatology implementation. Specifically, the key questions were:

KEY QUESTION #1

1a. How does the *accuracy* of teledermatology compare to usual care (in-person dermatology) for the *diagnosis* of skin conditions?

1b. How does the *concordance* of teledermatology compare to usual care (in-person dermatology) for the *diagnosis* of skin conditions?

KEY QUESTION #2

2a. How does the *accuracy* of teledermatology compare to usual care (in-person dermatology) for clinical *management* of skin conditions?

2b. How does the *concordance* of teledermatology compare to usual care (in-person dermatology) for clinical *management* of skin conditions?

KEY QUESTION #3

3. How do clinical outcomes (clinical course, satisfaction, quality of life, visits avoided) of teledermatology compare to usual care (in-person dermatology) for skin conditions?

KEY QUESTION #4

4. How does the cost of teledermatology compare to usual care (in-person dermatology)?

KEY QUESTION #5

5. What are the key structural and process elements associated with successful implementation of teledermatology and what are the barriers?

METHODS

We searched MEDLINE (OVID) and PubMed for controlled clinical trials, systematic reviews, cost studies, and implementation papers from 1990 to June, 2009 using standard search terms (Appendix A). We limited the search to peer-reviewed articles involving human subjects and published in English language. For key questions 1 and 2, inclusion was limited to controlled trials. Search terms included: remote consult/consultation, electronic mail, telecommunications, telemedicine, telepathology, dermatology, and teledermatology.

Titles and abstracts identified from the search were reviewed by physicians and research associates trained in the critical analysis of literature to identify peer-reviewed articles related to one or more of the key questions. We included studies of store and forward (SAF) and live interactive (LI) technologies.

Study characteristics, patient characteristics, and outcomes were extracted by a trained research associate under the supervision of the Principal Investigator, a Veterans Affairs (VA) dermatologist (Appendix B). We assessed study quality according to Quality Assessment of Diagnostic Accuracy Studies (QUADAS) criteria. We identified additional citations from reference lists of related articles. We performed pooled analyses where feasible and clinically appropriate. All other data were narratively summarized.

DATA SYNTHESIS

We constructed evidence tables showing study, patient, and intervention characteristics; methodological quality; and outcomes, organized by key question and teledermatology technology. We analyzed studies to compare their characteristics, methods, and findings. We compiled a summary of findings for each key question based on qualitative and semi-quantitative synthesis of the findings. Variability in patient, intervention, and outcome reporting limited pooling of findings across all studies, however, and when appropriate (similar technology and/ or skin conditions), weighted pooled averages were calculated. We identified and highlighted findings from VA or Department of Defense (DoD) populations.

PEER REVIEW

A draft version of this report was sent to two peer reviewers in addition to our Technical Expert Panel. Reviewer comments were addressed and our responses incorporated in the final report (Appendix C).

RESULTS
LITERATURE FLOW

The literature search yielded 658 citations, of which 185 articles met initial criteria for full-text level review. From these, we identified 85 references (including 69 controlled clinical trials) that addressed at least one of the key questions and met inclusion criteria. Among studies included to assess diagnostic accuracy and concordance (KQ1 and 2), most utilized methods to reduce sources of bias; particularly related to appropriate use of index and reference tests. However, the majority of studies using store and forward technology did not clearly address patient selection biases such as enrolling a representative spectrum of general dermatological patients or clearly describing exclusion criteria. Both store and forward and live interactive studies generally did not account for all patients at the end of the study or include patients with uninterpretable results.

OVERVIEW OF STUDIES FOR QUESTIONS 1 AND 2 (TABLE 2)

SAF: Forty-one SAF teledermatology studies met inclusion requirements and enrolled between 12 and 882 individuals. Of studies reporting specific subject characteristics, the mean age of enrollees was 53 years, 43% were female, and 93% were Caucasian. Twelve studies were conducted in the United States (5 involving veterans or military personnel). Eleven studies enrolled subjects specifically with pigmented lesions and one study enrolled subjects with non-pigmented lesions. Nineteen studies reported diagnostic accuracy (defined as a comparison of the diagnosis against histopathology/other laboratory test) and 27 studies reported diagnostic concordance (a comparison of the diagnoses made with teledermatology and clinical dermatology without verification by histopathology or laboratory test). Two studies reported management accuracy (a comparison of the teledermatology management plan against a management plan based on histopathology/other laboratory test) and 14 studies reported management concordance (a comparison of the management plans based on teledermatology and clinical dermatology).

LI: Ten LI teledermatology studies met inclusion requirements and enrolled between 51 and 351 individuals. The mean age of enrollees was 40 years, 54% were female, and 72% were Caucasian. Five of the studies were conducted in the United States and one study evaluated U.S. military personnel or veterans. One study enrolled subjects with isolated skin lesions; the remainder included subjects with both rashes and lesions. One LI study reported diagnostic accuracy, 10 reported diagnostic concordance, none reported management accuracy, and 4 reported management concordance.

Key Question #1a How does the accuracy of teledermatology compare to usual care (in-person dermatology) for the *diagnosis* of skin conditions? *(Table 3)*

Conclusion: Two-thirds of studies comparing teledermatology and usual care found better diagnostic accuracy with usual care (in-person dermatology visit) as compared to teledermatology. Estimates from subsamples of studies providing sufficient evidence for pooling suggested the magnitude of difference between the accuracy rates was approximately 11% and 19% for primary and aggregated diagnostic accuracy, respectively, and 5% for pigmented lesions. When dermatoscopy-trained teledermatologists were available, teledermatoscopy increased diagnostic accuracy of isolated skin lesions, although overall, rates were still not superior to usual care. One study found that the diagnostic accuracy of teledermatology was significantly worse for eleven common skin neoplasms including melanoma, squamous cell carcinoma, and basal cell carcinoma.

Summary of Studies: Twenty studies (19 SAF and 1 LI) reported diagnostic accuracy defined as matching of teledermatology diagnosis with histopathology diagnosis or other laboratory test. Results were reported as one or more of the following: 1) accuracy rate (percent match between the primary diagnosis and/or aggregated diagnoses [primary plus differential] and histopathology/laboratory test), 2) kappa statistic, and/or 3) sensitivity and specificity. Fifteen studies also assessed diagnostic accuracy of usual care (in-person dermatology diagnoses), allowing for direct comparisons between these two methods of care. Ten of these 15 studies reported better diagnostic accuracy for usual care (in-person dermatology visit) than teledermatology, 3 studies reported better accuracy for teledermatology, and 2 studies reported mixed results. Statistical pooling of the 6 SAF studies reporting aggregated diagnostic accuracy rates found that the weighted mean absolute difference between accuracy rates was 19% better for usual care than teledermatology. For the 11 SAF studies that reported primary diagnostic accuracy rates, the weighted mean absolute difference between accuracy rates was 11% better for usual care than teledermatology. Similarly, the weighted mean difference for primary diagnostic accuracy rates for six pigmented skin lesion studies was also better (5%) for usual care than teledermatology. Four studies evaluated teledermatology with standard macro images and teledermatoscopy. In general, teledermatology accuracy rates improved with teledermatoscopy (up to 15% absolute difference), although, overall, accuracy of teledermatoscopy was still not superior to usual care.

Key Question #1b How does the concordance of teledermatology compare to usual care (in-person dermatology) for the *diagnosis* of skin conditions? *(Table 4)*

Conclusion: Analysis from a limited subsample of studies providing sufficient evidence for pooling suggested that the aggregated diagnostic concordance rates for SAF teledermatology were similar for lesion studies (64%) and general studies (65%); the rate for LI (87%) was higher, but based on fewer patients. The weighted mean primary diagnostic concordance for SAF teledermatology was also similar for lesion studies (62%) and general studies (66%); the rate for LI studies was higher (71%) but based on fewer patients. In summary, diagnostic concordance of SAF was good and may be better for LI, possibly due to the ability to obtain additional history in the LI setting.

Summary of Studies: Thirty-seven (27 SAF, 9 LI, 1 SAF+LI) studies reported diagnostic concordance (simple agreement without verification by histopathology or laboratory test) between usual care (in-person dermatology visit) and teledermatology. Thirty-five studies (25 SAF, 9 LI, 1 SAF+LI) reported concordance as percent agreement for diagnosis, malignant/ benign status, or diagnostic category. Seven studies reported kappa statistics and three studies reported sensitivity and specificity.

Percent Concordance - SAF Studies: Weighted average diagnostic concordance rates for studies involving subjects with isolated skin lesions were 64% (aggregated, number of studies=4) and 62.3% (primary, n=6). Nineteen studies involving a range of dermatologic conditions (lesions and rashes) evaluated diagnostic concordance; rates ranged from 60-100% for aggregated diagnostic concordance (n=10) and 46-88% for primary diagnostic concordance (n=14). Excluding studies in which the same dermatologist served as both clinic dermatologist and teledermatologist, weighted average diagnostic concordance rates were 65% (aggregated, n=7) and 66% (primary, n=11).

Percent Concordance - LI Studies: Diagnostic concordance rates of LI ranged from 78-99% (aggregated, n=6) and 57-78% (primary, n=8). Excluding studies in which the same dermatologist served as both clinic dermatologist and teledermatologist, weighted average diagnostic concordance rates were 87% (aggregated, n=3) and 71% (primary, n=5).

Kappa, Sensitivity/Specificity: Kappa values ranged from 0.71-0.93 for the three SAF teledermatology studies reporting this statistic. Excluding the one study with likely bias (same dermatologist served as both clinic dermatologist and teledermatologist), kappa values indicated substantial agreement. Three LI studies reported kappa values that ranged from 0.32-0.79. Sensitivity and specificity was reported in three studies (utilizing the clinic dermatologist's assessment as the gold standard and agreement for benign or malignant status, not exact diagnosis). Sensitivity ranged from 0.88-1.0 and specificity ranged from 0.39-0.98.

Key Question #2a How does the accuracy of teledermatology compare to usual care (in-person dermatology) for clinical *management* of skin conditions? *(Table 5)*

Conclusion: While overall rates of management accuracy were equivalent (±10% absolute difference) for teledermatology and usual care, for malignant and premalignant lesions, rates for teledermatology and teledermatoscopy were inferior to usual care; caution is recommended when using teledermatology in these cases.

Summary of Studies: Only two studies, both by the same authors and using store and forward technology, evaluated management accuracy, defined as the percent agreement with an expert panel management plan based on histopathology. One study evaluated pigmented lesions and one evaluated non-pigmented lesions. The range for reported management accuracy was 70-80% for teledermatology compared to 66-84% for usual care. Clinical dermatology management accuracy rates were worse for pigmented lesions (66%) than non-pigmented lesions (84%).

Key Question #2b How does the concordance of teledermatology compare to usual care (in-person dermatology) for clinical *management* of skin conditions? *(Table 6)*

Conclusion: Concordance rates for management were moderate to excellent for both SAF and LI teledermatology (55-100%). The range for kappa statistic values was 0.47-0.71 (3 SAF studies and 1 LI) indicating fair to good agreement.

Summary of Studies:

SAF: Fifteen SAF teledermatology studies reported management concordance (percent agreement n=13, kappa n=3, sensitivity and specificity n=2). Two studies evaluated concordance of the triage management decision of "refer or not refer" for isolated skin lesions, yielding a weighted average rate of 75%. Two studies evaluated concordance rates for three different management options; these rates were 72% and 96%. Three studies evaluated concordance for the diagnostic procedure decision "biopsy or no biopsy" and found concordance rates of 76-100%. Several studies did not describe management options but reported percent concordance rates from 55-94%.

LI: Four LI teledermatology studies reported management concordance. The concordance rate for the decision "biopsy vs. no biopsy" for skin lesions was 86%. Three other studies involving a wide variety of skin conditions found concordance rates of 64%, 72%, and 75%.

Key Question #3 How do clinical outcomes (clinical course, satisfaction, quality of life, visits avoided) of teledermatology compare to usual care (in-person dermatology) for skin conditions? *(Tables 7, 8, and 9)*

Conclusion: There was insufficient evidence to conclude whether teledermatology had an effect on clinical course, although a large VA/DoD study reported comparable outcomes. Patient overall satisfaction with and preference for teledermatology or usual care were comparable in VA/DoD and other studies. Time to treatment was shorter and in-person visits can be avoided when patients are seen by teledermatology.

Summary of Studies: We identified 29 studies that reported clinical course, satisfaction, and/or visits avoided (17 SAF, 11 LI, and 1 SAF+LI). No studies reported quality of life. Among the SAF studies, two reported clinical course, nine reported patient satisfaction, and nine reported visits avoided. Three studies reported an additional outcome - time to treatment. Among the LI studies, one reported clinical course, nine reported patient satisfaction, and three reported visits avoided. The study that included both SAF and LI technologies reported only patient satisfaction.

Although two of three studies reporting clinical course suggested a more favorable outcome following teledermatology, these three studies used different methods for determining clinical course and assessed clinical course at different time points. The largest study, a VA and DoD study with over 500 patients, found no difference in the percentage of patient considered "improved" at 4 months after initial evaluation. Patients expressed comparable levels of satisfaction with teledermatology and usual care in three randomized, controlled trials (including one VA-based study). One non-randomized study reported greater satisfaction with teledermatology and one repeated measures study reported greater satisfaction with usual care. Response rates for the satisfaction assessments ranged from 58-100%. With the exception of one study which reported that 76% of subjects preferred teledermatology over waiting for a dermatology clinic appointment, preferences for teledermatology or usual care were similar. In one VA study, 42% preferred teledermatology over usual care while 37% preferred usual care over teledermatology. In five SAF studies that reported time to in-person consult or treatment, the time was shorter for patients who were initially seen by teledermatology. Teledermatology also reduced waiting times for clinic appointments and reduced the need for a in-person appointment by 14-66%.

Key Question #4 How does the cost of teledermatology compare to usual care (in-person dermatology)? *(Table 10)*

Conclusion: Cost analyses were limited by broad variations in cost assessment parameters and perspectives. Most studies found teledermatology to be cost effective if certain critical assumptions were met particularly patient travel distance, teledermatology volume, and the costs of usual care.

Summary of Studies: Three studies reported cost outcomes comparing SAF teledermatology to usual care. Six studies compared LI teledermatology to usual care. One study reported data from patients evaluated with both SAF and LI teledermatology. Wide differences existed in cost assessment parameters and perspectives evaluated (societal, health service, or patient). The majority of studies of SAF and LI found teledermatology to be cost effective if certain assumptions regarding patient travel distance, volume of teledermatology, and costs of usual dermatology care were met.

A micro-costing approach using a VA perspective found SAF teledermatology to be cost-effective, but not cost-saving, for decreasing time to initial definitive dermatologic care assuming that VA centers had both on-site primary care and dermatology clinics. The long-duration to achieve definitive dermatologic care, particularly for the usual care population (137.5 days vs. 50 days for the teledermatology group), however, is not consistent with current VA practice (all appointments within 30 days) and may result in an overly favorable estimate of teledermatology. A DoD study reported cost savings of $32 per patient if lost productivity was considered.

Key Question #5 What are the key structural and process elements associated with successful implementation of teledermatology and what are the barriers? *(Table 11)*

Conclusion: Key elements include: defining the setting for implementation, defining the objectives of the program, determining the organizational structure, identifying the resources available, considering all costs associated with teledermatology, determining the business model, procuring organizational support, and determining the training needs.

Summary of Studies: We attempted to categorize success facilitators using previously established definitions. We categorized implementation barriers according to administrative, clinical, patient, and technical factors. We emphasized factors likely to play a role in VA specific settings. We identified 12 descriptive studies that provided information relevant to implementation of a teledermatology program. Key elements included efficient and user-friendly programs, as well as ongoing technical and personnel support.

FUTURE RESEARCH RECOMMENDATIONS

Additional research is needed to determine the long-term effectiveness, feasibility, satisfaction, and cost-effectiveness of teledermatology, especially store and forward methodology. Standardized reporting of diagnostic, management, and outcome accuracy and concordance are important. Research evaluating clinical outcomes and patient management are especially needed. Studies that blind the assessor(s) to the patient/lesion/care method are preferred to reduce bias in outcome assessment. Additional outcomes could assess the impact of teledermatology on primary care practitioners' practice, satisfaction, and follow-up patterns. Barriers to successful implementation need to be identified that incorporate differences in patient populations, skin condition severity, distance traveled, availability of on-site dermatologists, and other clinical setting issues in order to determine the relative feasibility and effectiveness of different teledermatology strategies. Research priorities include comparing teledermatology with dermatologic care by a VA primary care provider or a dermatology trained nurse practitioner (rather than a dermatologist), assessing patient and primary care provider (as well as dermatologist) satisfaction with teledermatology, and conducting high quality cost effectiveness studies relevant to VA populations and care settings.

CONCLUSIONS

While the concordance of teledermatology and in-person dermatology care for diagnosis and management of skin conditions was generally acceptable, data from studies assessing accuracy indicate that accuracy of teledermatology is inferior to in-person dermatology care, especially for skin malignancies, an important and common condition in the veteran population. Little information exists on the impact of teledermatology on clinical outcomes. Patient and provider satisfaction with teledermatology were relatively high though there were individuals who have strong beliefs for a particular approach. Cost analysis studies were limited in number and relevance to current United States practice. Studies are needed to compare teledermatology with primary care to better understand the most effective way to deliver dermatology care in areas without reliable access to in-person dermatology (e.g., rural areas). . Given the results of this review, the potential benefits of teledermatology (e.g., decreased patient travel, shorter time to intervention, primary care provider education) need to be evaluated in the context of its limitations including inferior diagnostic accuracy and management accuracy, especially for malignant skin neoplasms.

INTRODUCTION AND BACKGROUND

Telemedicine uses telecommunication technology to transfer medical information. Due to the visual nature of a skin examination, telemedicine, specifically, teledermatology, is a potentially valuable tool in the diagnosis and management of dermatologic diseases for patients in rural areas (including rural Veterans Affairs Medical Centers [VAMCs] and Community Based Outpatient Clinics [CBOCs]) where a dermatologist may not be available. Teledermatology may also be useful in primary care settings to triage cases and limit unnecessary dermatology clinic referrals as well as to assist with follow-up care or monitoring after an in-person dermatology visit. Two particular types of teledermatology are commonly employed. Store and forward (SAF) uses asynchronous still digital image technology for communication, similar to an email system. Participants are typically separated by both time and space. Real-time or live interactive (LI) uses video-conferencing technology. Participants are separated by space, not by time. Both systems have advantages and disadvantages. SAF requires less technological sophistication and lower cost equipment than LI, permits the referring provider to submit the consultation with accompanying image(s) to the dermatologist for review at a later time, and does not require the dermatologist to be immediately available or on-call to urgently review the teleconsult while the patient is in the primary care clinic. In contrast, LI permits a more dynamic assessment of the skin condition and allows the dermatologist to obtain a real-time history from both the patient and the referring provider, to make an immediate initial diagnosis, and to provide a management plan. Owing partly to the technological simplicity of SAF and the fact that SAF allows the dermatologist to review the telemedicine consult either outside of normal clinic hours or bundled into separate time slots within an existing clinic, SAF is the more widely used form of teledermatology in the VA. An informal, unpublished survey of VA dermatology chiefs in December 2009 found that 44% (19/43) of responding VA dermatology services are utilizing teledermatology; 17 VAs are using SAF, one is using LI, and one is using both methodologies.

The diagnostic and management accuracy (match of teledermatology diagnosis or in-person dermatology diagnosis with a gold standard of histopathology or other laboratory test) and concordance (agreement between teledermatology and in-person dermatology) of these technologies, their cost-effectiveness, and their impact on clinical management and patient outcomes (including satisfaction) are not well understood. Although research demonstrating that teledermatology is accurate and cost-effective is essential, it is not sufficient. Lessons learned from mature, functioning teledermatology systems in the United Kingdom and New Zealand include that "initial concerns about the ability to diagnose and manage patients by telemedicine have turned out to be less important that the practical issues of implementation."[1] Incorporating research findings into clinical practice requires identifying and removing structural and process barriers as well as enhancing critical components to success. Based on the work of Rogers[2] and a systematic review of empirical research studies, Greenhalgh et al. developed a conceptual model for considering the determinants of diffusion, dissemination, and implementation of innovations in health service delivery and organization.[3] Greenhalgh et al. concluded that adoption of any health care technology increases to the degree that such technology is perceived as possessing the following qualities in relation to existing practice: *relative advantage* (the new technology is better than current processes); *compatibility* (consistency with existing values, behaviors and past experiences); *low complexity* (easy to understand and use); *trialability* (can be modified and experimented with on a limited basis), and *observability* (results of the change are visible).[3]

We conducted an evidence synthesis report to systematically review and summarize the scientific literature addressing: 1) teledermatology for the diagnosis of skin conditions, 2) teledermatology for the management of skin conditions, 3) clinical outcomes when teledermatology is used, 4) the cost of teledermatology compared with usual care (in-person dermatology), and 5) key elements of and barriers to successful implementation of teledermatology. We addressed the following key questions:

1a. How does the accuracy of teledermatology compare to usual care (in-person dermatology) for the *diagnosis* of skin conditions?

1b. How does the concordance of teledermatology compare to usual care (in-person dermatology) for the *diagnosis* of skin conditions?

2a. How does the accuracy of teledermatology compare to usual care (in-person dermatology) for clinical *management* of skin conditions?

2b. How does the concordance of teledermatology compare to usual care (in-person dermatology) for clinical *management* of skin conditions?

3. How do clinical outcomes (clinical course, satisfaction, quality of life, visits avoided) of teledermatology compare to usual care (in-person dermatology) for skin conditions?

4. How does the cost of teledermatology compare to usual care (in-person dermatology)?

5. What are the key structural and process elements associated with successful implementation of teledermatology and what are the barriers?

METHODS

TOPIC DEVELOPMENT, TECHNICAL EXPERT PANEL

This topic was nominated by the Center for Chronic Disease Outcomes Research, Minneapolis VA Medical Center in consultation with the VA Evidence Synthesis Program. Robert Dellavalle, MD, PhD; Dennis Oh, MD; and John Whited, MD, MHS agreed to serve on the Technical Expert Panel (TEP) for the project. The TEP and the VA Department of Health Services Research and Development (HSR&D) collaborated with the Minneapolis VA Evidence Synthesis Program (ESP) to identify and refine key questions including populations, interventions, comparisons, outcomes, and settings of relevance.

SEARCH STRATEGY

We searched MEDLINE (OVID) and PubMed for clinical trials, systematic reviews, cost studies, and implementation papers from 1990 to June, 2009 using standard search terms. We chose 1990 as the start date for the search based on consensus from the TEP members that studies prior to 1990 would likely not be relevant to current practice. We limited the search to articles involving human subjects and published in English language. Search terms included: remote consult/ consultation, electronic mail, telecommunications, telemedicine, telepathology, dermatology, and teledermatology. (Appendix A)

STUDY SELECTION

Titles and abstracts identified from the search were reviewed by physicians and research associates trained in the critical analysis of literature to identify peer-reviewed articles likely related to one or more of the key questions.

Specific inclusion criteria were as follows:

1. Controlled trial (questions 1 and 2)

2. Store and forward (SAF) or live interactive (LI) teledermatology

Specific exclusion criteria included:

1. Teledermatology involving mobile phones

2. Non-teledermatology settings (e.g., imaging analyses, telemedicine studies other than teledermatology, videomicroscopy studies, basic science, imaging techniques)

3. Dermatopathology studies

4. Reviews, teledermatology program descriptions, and history of teledermatology (unless

11

relevant to questions 3, 4 or 5)

5. Studies of computer-aided diagnoses only (e.g., pigmented lesions)

6. Survey studies addressing outcomes other than those defined in questions 1-5

7. Teledermatology as an educational tool for primary care physicians or residents

8. Technology assessment only

9. Remote monitoring of known diagnoses (e.g., leg ulcers, post-operative wounds)

10. Teledermatology involving patient generated photos and/or history (without a referring provider)

11. Non-English language

12. Case series with no control group (questions 1 and 2 only)

13. Commentaries, editorials or meeting abstracts (unless relevant to question 5)

14. Studies involving one diagnosis only (e.g., leprosy) or only acne and warts; studies of one category of skin conditions (e.g., pigmented lesions which could have multiple diagnoses) were included

15. Duplicate publications; if both preliminary and final reports were published, the final data analysis was utilized

16. Pediatric population only (as this would not be relevant to VA population); studies involving both adults and children were included.

For key questions 1 and 2 we included clinical trials of teledermatology with an in-person dermatology control group if they provided information related to diagnostic and management accuracy or concordance. For key question 3, we extracted data related to patient satisfaction and preferences. For key question 4 we obtained articles and evaluated past reviews assessing cost analyses of teledermatology programs with an emphasis on studies applicable to practice in the United States. For key question 5 we conducted a narrative review of identifiable information related to structural and process elements associated with successful implementation of teledermatology as well as barriers to implementation framing the section around the conceptual model developed by Greenhalgh et al.[3]

DATA ABSTRACTION

Two research associates (YH, NG) extracted data on study design, patient characteristics, lesion type(s), intervention(s), comparison(s), and outcome(s) from each included study for questions 1 to 4 (Appendix B – Data Extraction Form). The principal investigator verified all extracted data for these outcomes and also summarized data on implementation issues (question 5). Our main outcomes were diagnostic and management accuracy and concordance as defined in Table 1.

Table 1. Definitions of Outcomes

Outcome (Statistics Reported)	Definition
ACCURACY	**Match of TD (teledermatology) or CD (clinical dermatology) with Gold Standard of Histopathology or other Laboratory Test**
Diagnostic Accuracy – CD (% Correct, Kappa statistic, Sensitivity/Specificity)	Match of the CD diagnosis and histopathology/other lab test <u>Aggregated:</u> Match of any of the CD diagnoses (primary or differential diagnoses) with histopathology/lab diagnosis <u>Primary:</u> Match of the primary CD diagnosis with histopathology/lab diagnosis
Diagnostic Accuracy – TD (% Correct, Kappa statistic, Sensitivity/Specificity)	Match of the TD diagnosis and histopathology/ other lab test <u>Aggregated:</u> Match of any of the TD diagnoses (primary or differential diagnoses) with histopathology/lab diagnosis <u>Primary:</u> Match of the primary TD diagnosis with histopathology/lab diagnosis
Management Accuracy – CD (% Correct)	Match of the CD management plan with management based on histopathology/other lab test
Management Accuracy – TD (% Correct)	Match of the TD management plan with management based on histopathology/other lab test
CONCORDANCE	**Agreement between TD and CD**
Diagnostic Concordance (% Agreement, Kappa statistic)	Agreement between the TD diagnosis and the CD diagnosis <u>Aggregated:</u> Agreement of any of the TD diagnoses (primary or differential diagnoses) with any of the CD diagnoses (primary or differential diagnoses) <u>Primary:</u> Agreement of the primary TD diagnosis with the primary CD diagnosis
Management Concordance (% Agreement, Kappa statistic)	Agreement between the TD management and the CD management

QUALITY ASSESSMENT

We used the Quality Assessment of Diagnostic Accuracy Studies (QUADAS) instrument to assess for study quality for studies pertaining to key questions 1 and 2.[4] QUADAS is the first standardized, systematically developed, Delphi derived instrument used to assess methodological quality of studies of diagnostic tests. The QUADAS tool includes 14 questions that assess potential outcome bias. Items are scored as "yes," "no," or "uncertain" and can be grouped under 4 main domains: subject selection, index test, reference test, and data analysis. A summary score is not a recommended final metric of quality though we arbitrarily reported on the number of studies scored with a "yes" on at least 10 of 14 items as well the individual "yes" scores for each of the 4 domains. We believe such reporting can assist the reader in determining potential sources of study bias and encourage future researchers to adhere to these quality measures. Two extractors (EW, YH) independently reviewed all studies for quality. A third investigator (TW) resolved scoring discrepancies through review and discussion.

DATA SYNTHESIS

We reported results from each study separately for each outcome and method of outcome reporting (e.g., percent correct, kappa statistic, sensitivity/specificity, and concordance). Results were stratified according to whether the intervention was SAF or LI. We evaluated studies according to sample size, type of dermatological conditions studied, and whether they enrolled users of, and assessed outcomes in, the VA health care system. Due to considerable heterogeneity in study design, patient and lesion characteristics, and outcome reporting methods results were rarely pooled and instead displayed graphically according to teledermatology technology and sample size. If appropriate, weighted mean differences based on study sample sizes were calculated for the percentage of correct diagnoses for TD and usual care. Most pooled estimates were only possible using data from a subsample of eligible studies; caution is recommended in interpreting these pooled findings.

PEER REVIEW

A draft report was sent to TEP members and peer reviewers identified by VA HSR&D. Reviewer comments and author responses are summarized in Appendix C.

RESULTS

LITERATURE FLOW

The OVID MEDLINE search yielded 559 references with 3 duplicates for a total of 556 unique references. The PubMed search yielded 587 references. When the results from these searches were combined, 486 duplicate references were eliminated resulting in 657 titles and abstracts for review. From the 657 titles and abstracts, 473 references were excluded. The full text of 184 references was then reviewed and another 100 references were excluded. One additional reference (a recent publication) was added resulting in a total of 85 studies included in the report. Figure 1 details the exclusion criteria and the number of references related to each of the key questions.

KEY QUESTION 1

1a. How does the accuracy of teledermatology compare to usual care (in-person dermatology) for the *diagnosis* of skin conditions?

1b. How does the concordance of teledermatology compare to usual care (in-person dermatology) for the *diagnosis* of skin conditions?

Summary of Studies for Key Questions 1 and 2 (Table 2 and Appendix E)

The study design, population and study characteristics, teledermatology characteristics, outcomes evaluated, and the quality rating for each of the included studies are presented in Appendix E.

Description of store and forward studies

Study design and location

Forty-one unique store and forward studies (reported in 42 publications) enrolling between 12 and 882 subjects met inclusion criteria for Key Questions 1 and 2.[5,6,7,8,9,10,11,12,13,14,15,16,17,18,19,20,21,22,23,24,25,26,27,28,29,30,31,32,33,34,35,36,37,38,39,40,41,42,43,44,45,46] The majority of these studies each evaluated fewer than 200 subjects. All studies utilized a repeated measure study design with the exception of one randomized, controlled trial (RCT).[12] Based on location, most of the studies were conducted in the United States (n = 12),[5,6,7,23,25,26,34,36,38,42,43,44,46] followed by the United Kingdom (n = 9),[12,13,16,19,30,31,33,39,45] Italy, (n = 6),[8,9,21,22,37,40] Spain (n = 4),[10,11,14,18] Australia/New Zealand (n = 3),[15,32,41] Turkey (n = 2),[17,20] and one study each from Germany,[24] Netherlands,[25] Pakistan,[28] Brazil,[29] and Switzerland.[35]

Figure 1. Reference Flow Chart

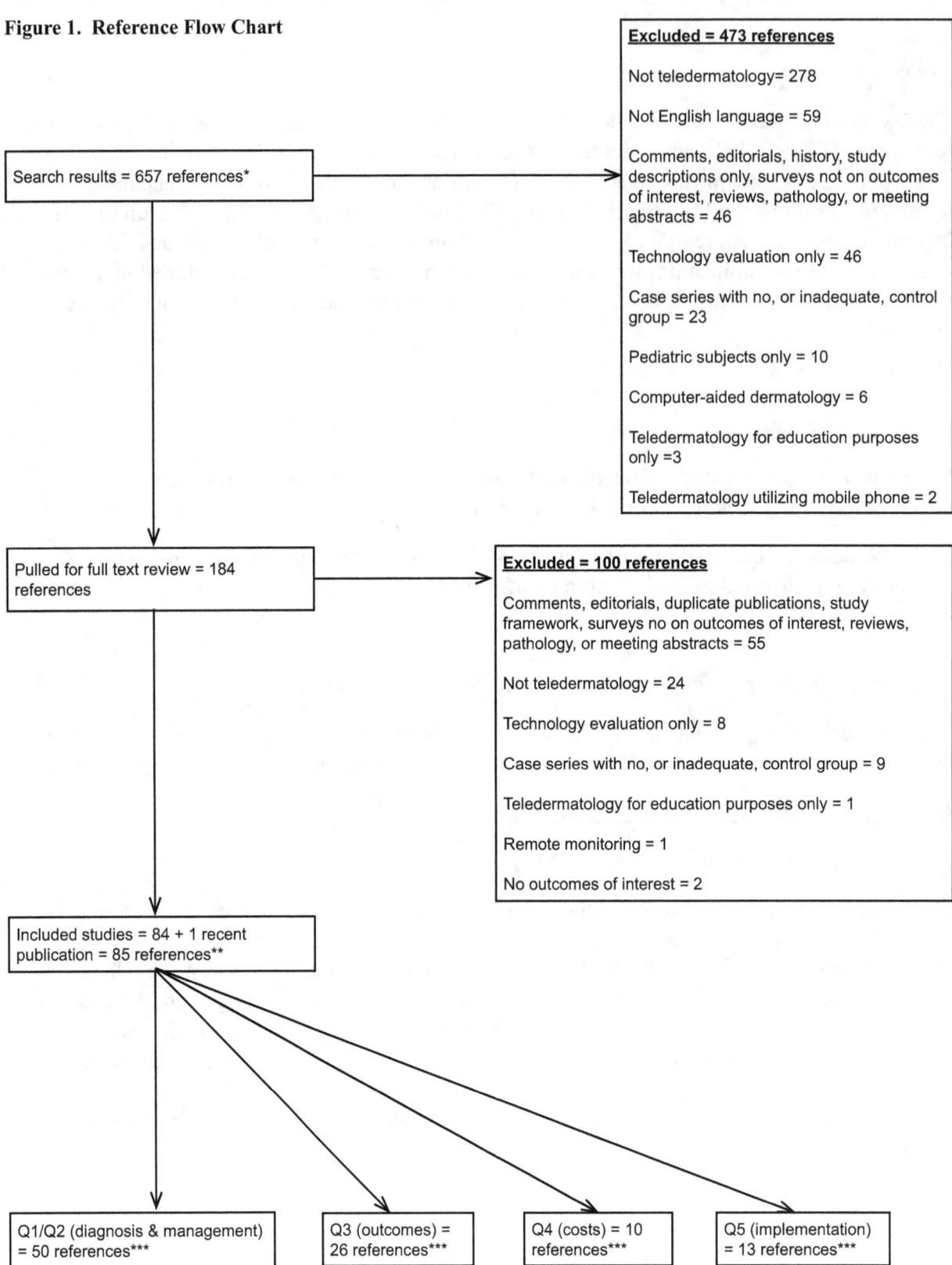

*Search results from OVID MEDLINE (556) and PubMed (587) were combined, removing duplicate entries (486)
**Manuscript reference list includes additional references cited for background and methods plus Web sites relevant to KQ5
***Total ≠ 85; many studies addressed more than one key question

Patient and skin condition characteristics

Five studies (six publications) involved U.S. military personnel and/or veterans.[5,6,26,27,42,43] The study by Pak also included beneficiaries of U.S. military personnel.[26,27] Fewer than half (19/41, 46.3%) of the studies reported mean age; of those reporting, mean age was 53 years (range of means 28 to 71 years). Thirteen studies included subjects less than 18 years of age, in addition to adults.[7,9,14,15,17,18,21,22,30,31,36,37,40] In 21 studies reporting gender, most of the subjects were male (57% overall, range 29% to 98%). Only 5 studies, all conducted in the United States, reported racial or ethnic characteristics.[5,6,7,26,27,42] The majority of subjects in those 5 studies were Caucasian (93%).

Fourteen studies included patients with a variety of skin conditions including rashes (e.g., papulosquamous, eczematous) as well as circumscribed lesions (isolated skin growths).[7,12,17,20,25,26,27, 28,32,33,36,38,42,45,46] Twenty-two studies evaluated only patients with circumscribed lesions (suspected skin cancer and/or isolated skin growths); of these, twelve studies exclusively evaluated subjects with pigmented skin lesions[5,9,14,18,21,22,24,30,31,35,37,40] and two studies enrolled only subjects with non-pigmented skin lesions.[6,8] The remaining eight studies only included subjects with circumscribed lesions but did not specify pigmentation status.[10,11,13,15,16,23,34,43] Five studies did not provide details on types of skin conditions included.[19,29,39,41,44]

Description of live interactive studies

Study design and location

Ten unique live interactive, repeated measure studies enrolling between 51 and 351 subjects met inclusion criteria for Key Questions 1 and/or 2.[7,17,47,48,49,50,51,52,43,54] Two of the studies also had a store and forward component.[7,17] One-half of the studies were conducted in the U.S. (n = 5).[7,49,51,52,54] Two studies were performed in the United Kingdom,[48,50] and one study each was completed in Turkey,[17] Norway,[47] and New Zealand.[53]

Patient and skin condition characteristics

One live interactive study involved U.S. veterans.[51] For the six studies reporting average age,[7,17,47,50,52,54] the mean age (40 years; mean range 35 to 47 years) was younger and less varied compared to the store and forward studies. Seven studies included children or adolescent subjects in addition to adults.[7,17,47,48,50,53,54] Three U.S. studies reported racial or ethnic characteristics,[7,51,54] overall, the majority of subjects in these three studies were Caucasian (72%), although the study by Lowitt included a significant number of African-American participants (40%).[51] Nearly all studies reported gender (n=9), with women comprising the majority of subjects (54%; mean range 5 to 84%).

Nine studies included patients with a variety of skin conditions including rashes (e.g., papulosquamous, eczematous) as well as circumscribed lesions (isolated skin growths).[7,17,47,48,49,5 0,51,53,54] One study evaluated only patients with circumscribed lesions (suspected skin cancer and/ or isolated skin growths).[52] No live interactive studies focused specifically on either pigmented or non-pigmented lesions.

Quality assessment

Most included studies assessing accuracy and concordance (Key Questions 1 and 2) utilized methods to reduce sources of bias, particularly related to appropriate use of index and reference tests. However, the majority of studies using store and forward technology did not clearly address patient selection biases such as enrolling a representative spectrum of general dermatological patients or clearly describing exclusion criteria. Both store and forward and live interactive studies generally did not account for all patients at the end of the study or include patients with uninterpretable results (**Figures 2 and 3**). Among individual studies, 11 of 41 SAF and 3 of 10 LI publications adequately reported on least 10 of 14 quality assessment items; most lower quality studies failed to adequately describe or enroll a representative spectrum of patients or account for all originally enrolled patients in data analysis.

QUESTION 1a: Diagnostic Accuracy (Table 3, Figures 4a and 4b)

Overall Comparisons: Twenty studies (19 SAF, 1 LI) reported diagnostic accuracy defined as matching of teledermatology diagnosis with histopathology diagnosis or other lab test. Results were reported as percent match between the primary diagnosis and/or aggregated diagnoses (primary plus differential) and histopathology, kappa statistic, and/or sensitivity and specificity. Fifteen studies also reported diagnostic accuracy of usual care (in-person dermatology diagnoses), allowing for direct comparisons of accuracy rates between these two methods of care. Ten of these 15 studies found that diagnostic accuracy for usual care (in-person dermatology visit) was better than teledermatology,[5,6,8,15,24,34,37,38,40,42] 3 studies reported better diagnostic accuracy for teledermatology,[30,35,51] and 2 reported mixed results.[26,27,43] The three studies which reported higher diagnostic accuracy rates for teledermatology were comprised of smaller sample sizes (n=11,[51] n=51,[35] n= 138[30]). In the small pilot study by Lowitt[51] the difference between accuracy rates was the result of one lesion, a difference likely due to chance. In the study by Braun[35] involving 55 pigmented skin lesions in 51 patients, diagnoses were compared between six general dermatologists in private practice (usual care) with a dermatoscopic expert at a university pigmented skin lesion clinic (teledermatologist). The better diagnostic accuracy of the teledermatologist in this study was likely due to dermatoscopic expertise; the six general dermatologists had "different levels of experience" whereas the teledermatologist was a dermatoscopic expert. In the larger study by Jolliffe[31] involving 144 pigmented skin lesions in 138 patients, the same dermatologist who saw the patient in clinic (and likely followed up on biopsy results) served as teledermatologist (several months later), possibly resulting in recall bias.

Pooled Comparisons: Statistical pooling of the six SAF studies reporting aggregated diagnostic accuracy rates found that the weighted mean absolute difference was 19% better for usual care than teledermatology.[5,6,26,27,34,42,43] For the 11 SAF studies[5,6,15,24,26,27,30,35,37,40,42,43] which reported primary diagnostic accuracy rates, the weighted mean absolute difference was 11% better for usual care than teledermatology. Similarly, the weighted mean absolute difference for primary diagnostic accuracy for six pigmented skin lesion studies was also better (5%) for usual care than teledermatology.[5,24,30,35.37,40] A recent unpublished analysis of teledermatology data from 1514 biopsied skin neoplasms found that teledermatology was significantly less accurate for eleven common skin neoplasms including melanoma, squamous cell carcinoma, and basal cell carcinoma.[55]

Value of Teledermatoscopy: Four studies evaluated teledermatology with standard macro images and teledermatoscopy.[5,6,8,14] In general, teledermatology accuracy rates improved up to 15% (absolute difference) with teledermatoscopy. A recent unpublished analysis found that diagnostic accuracy significantly improved with polarized light teledermatoscopy specifically for squamous cell carcinoma and basal cell carcinoma.[55]

Conclusion: The evidence shows that diagnostic accuracy of usual care (in-person dermatology) is better than teledermatology (aggregated diagnostic accuracy absolute difference 19%; primary diagnostic accuracy absolute difference 5% and 11%). When dermatoscopy-trained teledermatologists are available, teledermatoscopy may be beneficial for isolated skin lesions.

QUESTION 1b: Diagnostic Concordance (Table 4, Figures 5a, 5b, 6a and 6b)

Overall Comparisons: Thirty-seven (27 SAF; 9 LI; 1 SAF+LI) studies reported diagnostic concordance (simple agreement without verification by histopathology or laboratory test) between usual care (in-person dermatology) and teledermatology. Thirty-five studies (25 SAF, 9 LI, 1 SF+LI) reported concordance as percent agreement for exact diagnosis (primary-*see figures 5b and 6b*, aggregated-*see figures 5a and 6a*, and/or not specified,[7,45,46] malignant/benign status,[13,29,39] or diagnostic category.[51] Seven studies in six publications reported kappa statistics[7,11,18,29,52,53] and three studies reported sensitivity and specificity.[13,29,39]

Percent Concordance - SAF Lesion Study Results: Aggregated diagnostic agreement was assessed in 4 studies (Table 4, Figure 5a). Two medium-sized studies, both of which evaluated circumscribed skin lesions, found similar aggregated diagnostic concordance rates of 64% (n=109[15]) and 65% (n=163[16]). Two smaller lesion studies found higher aggregated diagnostic concordance rates, 90% (n=50[34]) and 95% (n=10[43]). Weighted average aggregated diagnostic concordance of these four lesion studies was 64.4% (230/358). Primary diagnostic concordance (Table 4, Figure 5b) was assessed in one pigmented lesion study[40] and five skin lesion studies;[13,15,16,34,43] concordance ranged from 48% to 91%. Weighted average for these six studies was 62.3% (443/708).

Percent Concordance - SAF General Study Results: Nineteen studies involving a range of dermatologic conditions (lesions and rashes) evaluated diagnostic concordance (Table 4, Figures 5a and 5b). Aggregated diagnostic agreement was assessed in ten of these studies and ranged from 60-100%. The three highest rates were from studies in which the same dermatologist served as both clinic dermatologist and teledermatologist and did not appear to be blinded to index results (91%,[26,27] 96%,[32] and 100%[41]). Excluding those three studies, the weighted average aggregated diagnostic agreement rate was 65.3% (703/1077). Primary diagnostic agreement was assessed in 14 studies and ranged from 46% to 88%. Excluding the three studies where the same dermatologist served as both clinic dermatologist and teledermatologist (70%,[26,27] 88%,[32] and 83%[41]), the weighted average primary diagnostic concordance rate was 66.3% (1227/1851).

Percent Concordance - LI Studies: Six LI studies reported aggregated diagnostic concordance rates ranging from 78 to 99% (Figure 6a); excluding three studies in which the same dermatologist served as both clinic dermatologist and teledermatologist for >50% of cases (78%,[48] 82%,[53] 82%[50]), the weighted average aggregated diagnostic concordance was 86.5% (268/310). Eight LI studies reported primary diagnostic concordance rates ranging from 57-

78% (Figure 6b); excluding three studies in which the same dermatologist served as both clinic dermatologist and teledermatologist (67%,[48] 75%,[53] 67%[50]), the weighted average primary diagnostic concordance rate was 70.5% (258/366).

Kappa, Sensitivity, Specificity

SAF Studies: Kappa values ranged from 0.71 to 0.93 for the four SAF teledermatology studies reporting this statistic.[7,11,18,29] Excluding the one study with likely bias (same dermatologist served as both clinic dermatologist and teledermatologist, k=0.93[18]), kappa values varied by 16 points and values indicated substantial agreement (k=0.71,[7] k=0.81,[11] k=0.87[29]). Sensitivity and specificity was reported in three studies (utilizing the clinic dermatologist's assessment as the gold standard); all three evaluated only agreement for benign or malignant status, not specific diagnosis. Sensitivity ranged from 0.88 to 1.0 and specificity ranged from 0.39 to 0.98.

LI Studies: Three LI studies reported kappa values of 0.32,[52] 0.62,[53] and 0.79.[7] The study by Phillips[52] had the lowest kappa value (k=0.32); this study employed a live interactive system which may not have been able to provide the detail required for the individual skin lesions evaluated. No LI studies evaluated sensitivity or specificity.

LI+SAF Study Results: Only one study evaluated a combination of SAF and LI teledermatology.[17] In that study, primary diagnostic accuracy concordance was 82%, higher than the weighted average concordance rate of SAF studies (66.3%) and LI studies (70.5%).

Conclusion: Based on the data above, the weighted mean aggregated diagnostic concordance rates for SAF teledermatology were similar for lesion studies (64%) and general studies (65%); the rate for LI (87%) was higher, but this was based on significantly fewer patients (approximately 300 vs. >1,000). The weighted mean primary diagnostic concordance for SAF teledermatology was also similar for lesion studies (62%) and general studies (66%); the rate for LI studies was higher (71%) but based on fewer patients. In summary, diagnostic concordance of SAF is good and may be better for LI, possibly due to the ability to obtain additional history in the LI setting.

KEY QUESTION 2

QUESTION 2a. How does the accuracy of teledermatology compare to usual care (in-person dermatology) for clinical *management* of skin conditions? (Table 5)

Only two studies assessed management accuracy (expert panel consensus of management based on histopathologic diagnosis) of usual care and teledermatology.[5,6] Both were large, utilized SAF teledermatology, were completed at the same VA, enrolled primarily older, Caucasian, men, and involved circumscribed skin lesions. In both studies, overall management was equivalent (defined as a ±10% difference) for usual care and teledermatology (macro images as well as two types of dermatoscopic images). Although the overall management accuracy rates were not significantly different, further unpublished analysis of this data provided by the lead author of this evidence report found that nine melanomas were mismanaged with teledermatology as compared to two with usual care, and management accuracy of usual care was superior to teledermatology (macro images or dermatoscopic images) not only for melanoma but also for basal cell carcinoma, squamous cell carcinoma, and premalignant actinic keratoses.[55]

Conclusion: While overall rates of management accuracy were equivalent (±10%), for malignant and premalignant lesions, rates for teledermatology and teledermatoscopy were inferior to usual care; caution is recommended when using teledermatology in these cases. Because only two studies reported management accuracy, these results may be difficult to generalize to other populations and study settings.

QUESTION 2b. How does the concordance of teledermatology compare to usual care (in-person dermatology) for clinical *management* of skin conditions? (Table 6, Figures 7a and 7b)

SAF Studies: Fourteen SAF teledermatology studies reported management concordance (percent agreement n=13, kappa n=3, sensitivity and specificity n=2).[7,9,10,12,13,15,16,23,26,31,42,43,45,46] Two studies evaluated concordance of the triage management decision of "refer or not refer" for pigmented skin lesions[31] or skin lesions;[13] percent concordance was 80%[31] and 61%[13] for these two studies yielding a weighted average of 75.3% (809/1075). Three studies (in four publications) evaluated concordance for the diagnostic procedure decision "biopsy or no biopsy" and found concordance rates of 100%[23] and 95%[43] for skin lesions (weighted average of 98.5%, 68/69) and 76% for a variety of skin conditions.[26,27] Several studies did not describe management options but reported percent concordance rates of 55% to 94% (Figure 7a).[7,12,15,16,45,46] Two studies evaluated concordance rates for three different management options; these rates were 96%[9] and 72%.[42]

Three studies reported the following kappa statistics: k=0.69 for three management options for 265 pigmented skin lesions in 18 patients;[9] k=0.75 for planned surgical technique for 134 skin lesions;[10] and k=0.62 for 110 skin conditions.[7] Sensitivity/specificity ranged from 0.69/0.82 (refer or not refer[31]) to 1.0/1.0 (biopsy or no biopsy[23]).

LI Studies: Four LI teledermatology studies reported management concordance.[7,48,52,56] A study of 107 skin lesions in 51 patients found a concordance rate of 86% (k=0.47) for the decision "biopsy or no biopsy."[52] Three other studies involving a wide variety of skin conditions found concordance rates of 64%,[56] 72%,[48] and 75%.[7] No LI studies reported sensitivity/specificity.

Conclusion: Concordance rates for management were moderate to very good for both SAF and LI teledermatology.

Table 2. Summary of Study Characteristics for Teledermatology Studies (KQ1 and KQ2)

Characteristic	Store and Forward (N=41)		Live Interactive (N=10)	
	Mean and/or Range	Number of Studies Reporting	Mean and/or Range	Number of Studies Reporting
Number of Subjects: Repeated measure studies	12 to 882 (NR in 3)	40	51 to 351	10
Randomized controlled trials (TD arm only)	92	1	NA	0
Studies involving US Military Personnel or Veterans: Number of subjects	129 to 728	5	102	1
Age of Subjects in Years: All studies, weighted mean (mean range)	53 (28 to 71)	19	40 (35 to 47)	6
Studies with children/adolescents (<18 years of age) in addition to adults	NR	13	NR	7
Gender: Female: mean % (mean range)	43 (2 to 71)	21	54 (5 to 84)	9
Race: Caucasian: mean % (mean range)	93 (80 to 99)	5	72 (60 to 85)	3
Black: mean % (mean range)	5 (12 to 20)	5	27 (12 to 40)	3
Other: mean % (mean range)	2 (<1 to 5)	5	1 (0 to 3)	3
Study Location in U.S: Number of subjects per study	12 to 728	12	51 to 131	5
Skin Condition Characteristics: Rashes and lesions number of subjects per study	23 to 404	14	60 to 351	9
Lesions only number of subjects per study	12 to 882 (NR in 2)	22	51	1
Pigmented lesions only number of subjects per study	12 to 611 (NR in 1)	12	NA	0
Non-pigmented lesions only number of subjects per study	728 (NR in 1)	2	NA	0
Outcomes Assessed: Diagnostic accuracy number of subjects per study	12 to 728	19	102	1
Diagnostic concordance number of subjects per study	12 to 882	27	51 to 351	10
Management accuracy number of subjects per study	542 to 728	2	NA	0
Management concordance number of subjects per study	12 to 882	14	51 to 351	4

Figure 2.

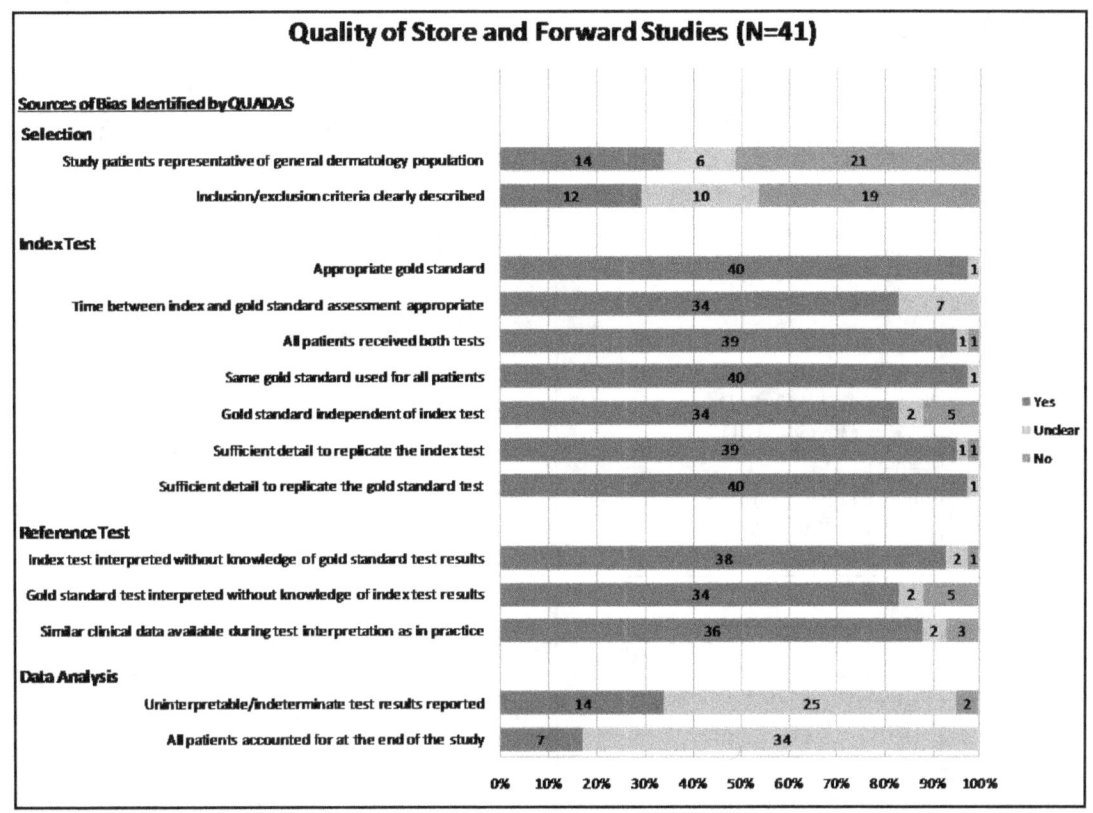

Figure 3.

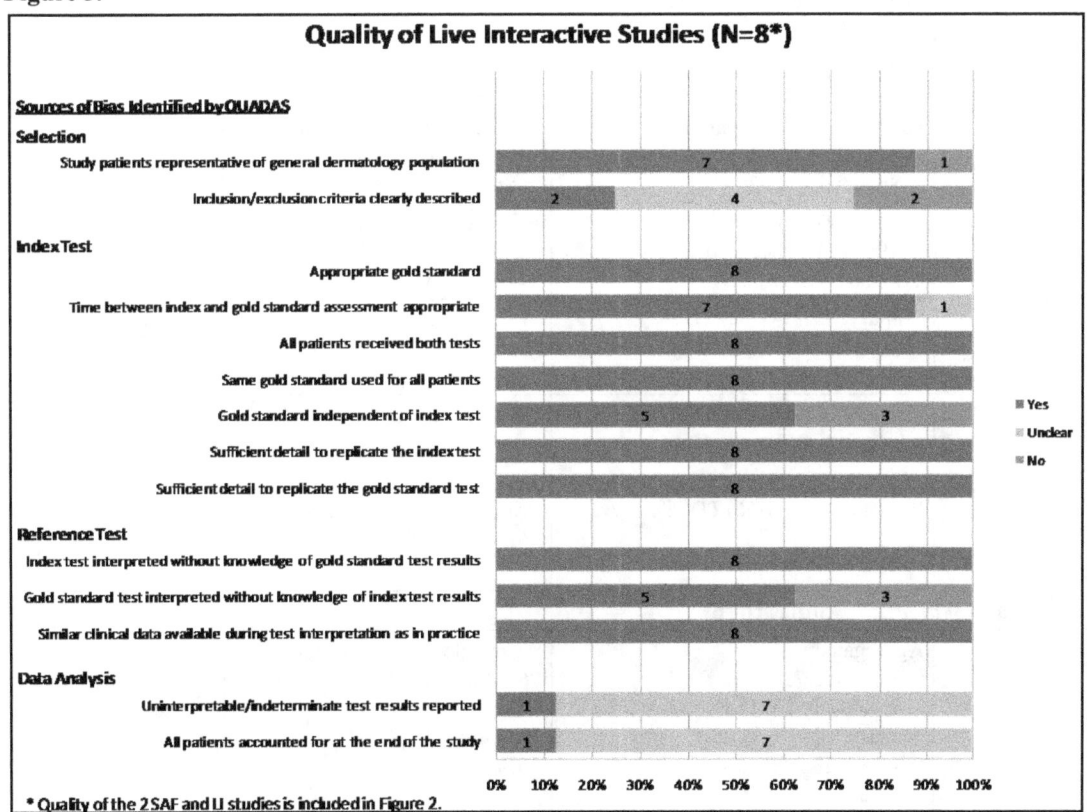

* Quality of the 2 SAF and LI studies is included in Figure 2.

Table 3. Studies Reporting Diagnostic Accuracy using Histopathology/Lab Tests as Gold Standard (KQ1a) (See Appendix D for abbreviations)

Study	Diagnostic Accuracy - Teledermatology % Correct, Kappa, or Sensitivity/Specificity	Diagnostic Accuracy - Usual Care % Correct, Kappa, or Sensitivity/Specificity	Mean Absolute Difference, % Correct
A. Store and forward *pigmented skin lesion* studies (n=10)			
Warshaw 2009[5] VA 542 Pts 542 PSL	Aggregated: 52% (282/542) 65% (352/542) PLD 67% (363/542) CID Primary: 50% (271/542) 47% (255/542) PLD 57% (309/542) CID	Aggregated: 80% (434/542) Primary: 59% (320/542)	-28% -9%
Moreno-Ramirez 2006[14] 61 Pts No. PSL NR	k=0.91 (95% CI 0.82, 1.00) k=0.94 TDSC (95% CI 0.88, 1.00)	NR	NA
Moreno-Ramirez 2005[18] No. Pts NR 57 PSL	k=0.79 (95% CI 0.70, 0.89)	NR	NA
Ferrara 2004[21] 12 Pts 12 PSL	Primary: 83% (10/12) TDSC	NR	NA
Piccolo 2004[22] 73 Pts 77 PSL	Mean Sensitivity for 11 TDs: 0.91 (SD 0.09) (Range 0.83-1.00) Mean Specificity for 11 TDs: 0.95 (SD 0.04) (Range 0.92-1.00)	NR	NA
Coras 2003[24] No. Pts NR 45 PSL	Primary: 89% (40/45) TDSC For Malignant vs. Benign: Sensitivity: 0.86 Specificity: 0.92	Primary: 91% (41/45) DSC For Malignant vs. Benign: Sensitivity: 0.86 Specificity 0.96	-2%
Jolliffe 2001[30] 138 Pts 144 PSL	Primary: 47% (68/144) (95% CI 39%, 55%) TD also served as CD	Primary: 43% (63/144) (95% CI 35%, 51%) TD also served as CD	4%
Braun 2000[35] 51 Pts 55 PSL	Primary: 75% (41/55) TDSC	Primary: 64% (35/55) DSC	11%
Piccolo 2000[37] 40 Pts 43 PSL	Primary: 87% avg for 6 derms TDSC (range 81%-95%)	Primary: 91% (39/43) DSC	-4%
Piccolo 1999[40] 66 Pts 66 PSL	Primary 86% (57/66) TDSC	Primary 92% (61/66) DSC	-6%
B. Store and forward *skin lesion* studies (n=6)			
Warshaw 2009[6] VA 728 Pts 728 SL	Aggregated: 56% (408/728) 65% (473/728) PLD Primary: 43% (313/728) 47% (342/728) PLD	Aggregated: 76% (553/728) Primary: 56% (408/728)	-20% -13%

Fabbrocini 2007[8] No. Pts NR 44 SL	k=0.44 k=0.45 CID	k=0.52 k=0.70 CID	NA
Ferrandiz 2007[10] 134 Pts No. SL NR (73% NMSC)	Primary: 85% (110/130) k=0.86 (95% CI 0.83, 0.89)	NR	NA
Oakley 2006[15] No. of Pts NR 29 SL	Primary: 71% (34/48) (95% CI 56, 83) 38 TDs including 6 residents	Primary: 72% (21/29) (95% CI 53, 87%) 5 CDs including 2 plastic surgeons	-1%
Barnard 2000[34] 25 "cases"	Aggregated: 73% avg for 8TDs (range 54%-80%)	Aggregated: 84%	-11%

Whited 1998[43]
VA
9 SL
	Aggregated average: 84%
	    Aggregated (2 TDs):
	89% (8/9)
	78% (7/9)
	Primary average: 59%
	    Primary (2 TDs):
	78% (7/9)
	22% (2/9)
		Aggregated: 78% (7/9)
		
		Primary: 67% (6/7)
			6%
			
			-8%

C. Store and forward *general* studies (n=3)			
Pak 2003 (part II)[26] DoD 119 Pts 119 Conditions	Aggregated: 78% (No. NR) Primary 19%	Aggregated: 60% Primary: 73%	18% -54%
Krupinski 1999[38] 104 Pts 104 Conditions	Primary: 76% Avg for 3 TDs	Primary/Aggregated: 89% Avg for 3 CDs (Combo 58% Primary; 42% Aggregated)	-13%

Whited 1999[42]
VA
No. Pts NR
79 Conditions
	Aggregated average: 77%
	    Aggregated (3 TDs):
	68% (95% CI 58%, 78%)
	78% (95% CI 69%, 87%)
	85% (95% CI 77%, 93%)
	Primary average: 59%
	    Primary (3 TDs):
	53% (95% CI 42%, 64%)
	63% (95% CI 52%, 74%)
	62% (95% CI 51%, 73%)
		Aggregated: 85% (95% CI 77%,
		93%)
		
		Primary: 59% (95% CI 48%,
		70%)
			-8%
			
			0

Weighted mean difference for aggregated diagnosis studies (range of mean differences; # studies)	**-19% (-28 to 18%; 6 studies)[5,6,26,34,42,43]**		
Weighted mean difference for primary diagnosis studies (range of mean differences; # studies)	**-11% (-54 to 11%; 11 studies)[5,6,15,24,26,30,35,37,40,42,43]**		
Weighted mean difference for primary diagnosis *pigmented skin lesion* studies (range of mean differences; # studies)	**-5% (-9 to 11%; 6 studies)[5,24,30,35,37,40]**		
D. Live interactive studies (n=1)			
Lowitt 1998[51] VA No. Pts NR 11 Conditions	Aggregated: 73% (8/11)	Aggregated: 64% (7/11)	9%

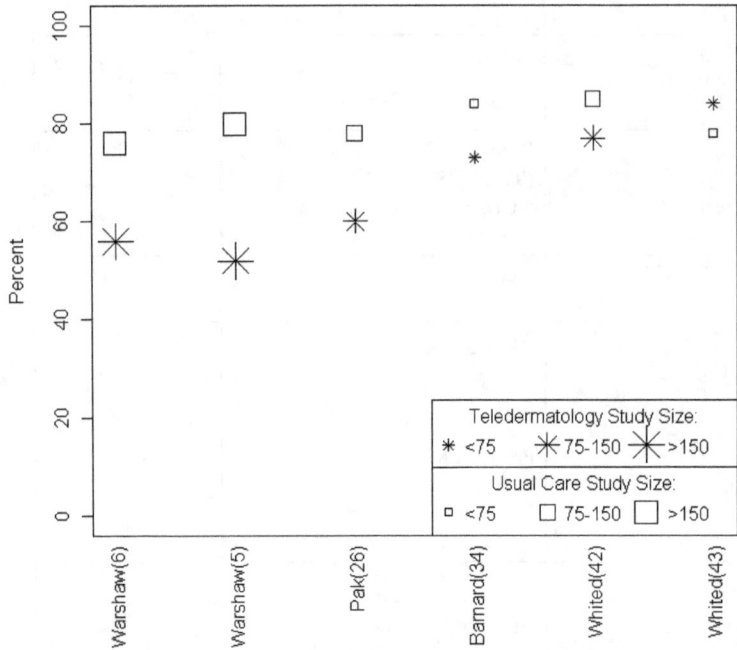

Figure 4a

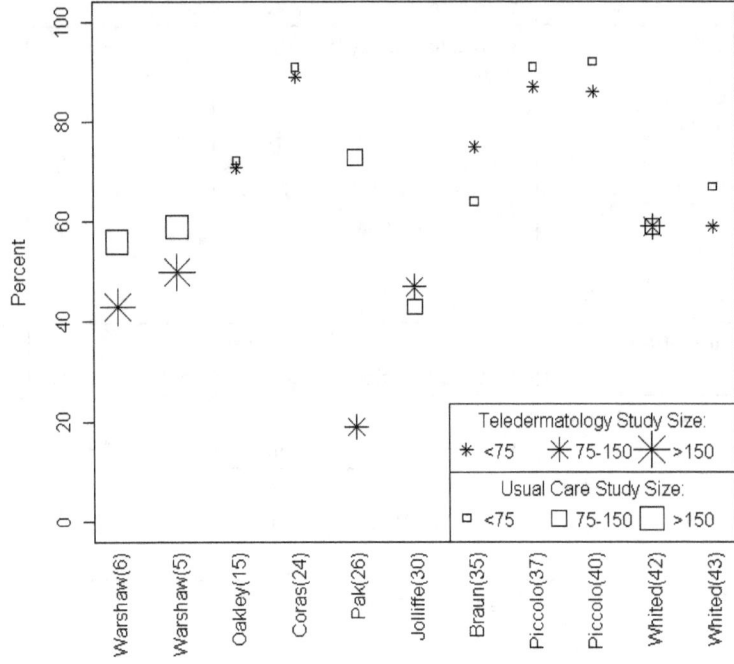

Figure 4b.

Table 4. Studies for Reporting Diagnostic Concordance between Teledermatology and Usual Care (In-Person Dermatology) (KQ1b)*

Study No. of subjects No. of skin conditions	Percent concordant	Kappa statistic	Sensitivity and Specificity
A. Store and forward *pigmented skin lesion* studies (n=2)			
Moreno-Ramirez 2005[18] 108 Pts No. PSL NR	NR	k=0.93 (95% CI 0.87, 0.98) TD = CD	NR
Piccolo 1999[40] 66 Pts 66 PSL	Primary: 91% (60/66) *DSC*	NR	NR
B. Store and forward *skin lesion* studies (n=6)			
Moreno-Ramirez 2007[11] 882 Pts 882 SL	NR	k=0.81 (95% CI 0.78, 0.84)	NR
Bowns 2006[13] 256 Pts 256 SL	Primary: 69% (159/230) agreement on specific diagnosis TDSC: 75% (193/256) agreement on benign or malignant	NR	TD: Sensitivity=0.98 (95% CI 0.92, 0.99) Specificity= 0.39 (95% CI 0.32, 0.47) TDSC: Sensitivity=0.98 (95% CI 0.92, 0.99) Specificity=0.43 (95% CI 0.36, 0.51)
Oakley 2006[15] 73 Pts 109 SL	Aggregated: 64%, No. NR Primary: 53% (100/189) (95% CI 46, 60%) *TD=38 dermatologists including residents* *CD=3 dermatologists and 2 plastic surgeons*	NR	NR
Mahendran 2005[16] 163 Pts 163 SL	Aggregated: 65% (106/163) Primary: 48% (78/163)	NR	NR
Barnard 2000[34] 50 "cases"	Aggregated: 90%, No. NR (range for 8TDs 86-96%) Primary: 77%, No. NR (range for 8 TDs 67%-84%)	NR	NR
Whited 1998[43] VA 12 Pts 10 SL	2TDs - Aggregated: 90% (9/10) 100% (10/10) Primary: 80% (8/10) 60% (6/10)	NR	NR
C. Store and forward *general* studies (n=19)			
Edison 2008[7] 110 Pts 110 Conditions	Primary: 73% (80/110) (95% CI 64, 81%)	k=0.71 (95% CI 0.67, 0.76)	NR
Bowns 2006[12] 92 Pts 92 Conditions	Primary: 55% (51/92)	NR	NR

Baba 2005[17]
228 Pts
242 Conditions
	Primary:
	  TD also served as CD: 81% (197/242)
	  TD not the same as CD: 75% (181/242)
		NR	NR

Tucker 2005[19] 75 Pts 84 Conditions	Aggregated: 68% (57/184) Primary: 56% (47/84)	NR	NR
Oztas 2004[20] 125 Pts 125 Conditions	Primary: 70% (88/125) Average of 3 TDs	NR	NR
Du Moulin 2003[25] 106 Pts 106 Conditions	Aggregated: 63% (67/106) Primary: 54% (57/106)	NR	NR
Pak 2003[27] DoD 404 Pts 404 Conditions	Aggregated: 91% (366/404) Primary: 70% (283/404) TD also served as CD (included residents)	NR	NR
Rashid 2003[28] 33 Pts 33 Conditions	Aggregated: 81% (27/33)	NR	NR
Oliveira 2002[29] 92 Pts No. Conditions NR	98% (88/90) for benign vs. malignant	k=0.87	Sensitivity=1.00 Specificity=0.98
Lim 2001[32] 23 Pts 27 Conditions	Aggregated: 96%, No. NR Primary: 88%, No. NR TD also served as CD	NR	NR
Taylor 2001[33] 188 Pts No. of Conditions NR	Aggregated: 60%, No. NR Primary: 50%, No. NR	NR	NR

High 2000[36]
92 Pts
106 Conditions
	Aggregated:
	  85% (84/99)
	  64% (49/77)
	  77% (76/99)
	Primary:
	  70% (69/99)
	  64% (49/77)
	  77% (76/99)
		NR	NR

Krupinski 1999[38]
308 Pts
308 Conditions
	3 TDs (some also served as CD)
	Primary:
	  81%, No. NR
	  84%
	  85%
	Average of all 3: 83%
		NR	NR

Lewis 1999[39] 56 Cases	93% No. NR (likelihood of benign vs. malignant on 1-5 scale)	NR	Sensitivity=0.88 Specificity=0.80 *(benign vs. malignant)*
Tait 1999[41] 30 Pts No. of Conditions NR	Aggregated: 100% (30/30) Primary: 83% (25/30) TD also served as CD	NR	NR

Whited 1999[42]
VA
129 Pts
168 Conditions
	3 TDs - Aggregated:
	  84% (95% CI 79%, 90%)
	  83% (95% CI 78%, 89%)
	  95% (95% CI 92%, 98%)
	Primary:
	  41% (95% CI 34%, 49%)
	  44% (95% CI 36%, 52%)
	  52% (95% CI 45%, 60%)
	Average = 46%
		NR	NR

Kvedar 1997[44]
No. of Pts NR
123 Conditions
	2 TDs - Aggregated:
	  70%
	  67%
	Primary:
	  61%
	  64%
		NR	NR

Lyon 1997[45] 100 Pts 100 Conditions	93% (93/100) TD staff; CD resident	NR	NR
Zelickson 1997[46] 29 Pts 30 Conditions	88% (53/60) Combination of 2-3 TDs	NR	NR
D. Live interactive studies *skin lesion* studies (n=1)			
Phillips 1998[52] 51 Pts 107 SL	Primary: 59% (63/107)	k=0.32	NR
E. Live interactive *general* studies (n=8)			
Edison 2008[7] 110 Pts 110 Conditions	80% (88/110) (95% CI 73%, 88%)	k=0.79 95% CI 0.75, 0.83)	NR
Nordal 2001[47] 112 Pts 112 Conditions	Aggregated: 86% (97/112) Primary: 72% (81/112)	NR	NR
Gilmour 1998[48] 126 Pts 155 Conditions	Aggregated: 78% (121/155) Primary: 57% (88/155) TD also served as CD in 51% (79/155) of cases	NR	NR
Lesher 1998[49] 60 Pts 68 Conditions	Aggregated: 99% (67/68) Primary: 78% (53/68)	NR	NR
Loane 1998[50] 351 Pts 427 Conditions	Aggregated: 82% (352/427) Primary: 67% (285/427) TD also served as CD in 63% (226/427) of cases	NR	NR
Lowitt 1998[51] VA 102 Pts 130 Conditions	Aggregated: 80% (104/130) Agreement for diagnostic category	NR	NR
Oakley 1997[53] 104 Pts 135 Conditions	Aggregated: 82% (110/135) Primary: 75% (101/135) TD also served as CD in 79% of cases	k=0.62 (TD not the same as CD) k=0.91 (TD also served as CD)	NR
Phillips 1997[54] 60 Pts 79 Conditions	Primary: 77% (61/79)	NR	NR
F. Live interactive and store and forward studies (n=1)			

Baba 2005[17]
228 Pts
242 Conditions
	Primary:
	  90% (218/242) TD also served as CD
	  82% (199/242) TD not the same as CD
		NR	NR

*Results for staff dermatologists unless otherwise reported.

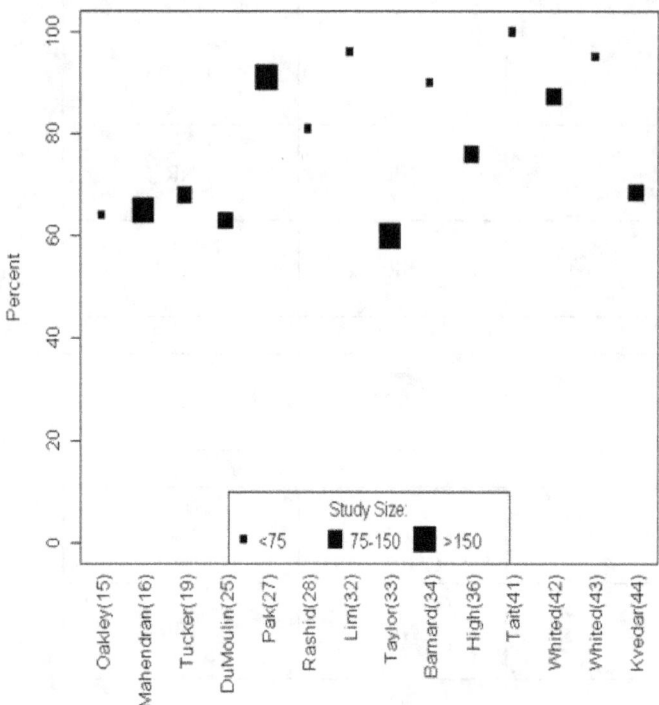

Figure 5a.

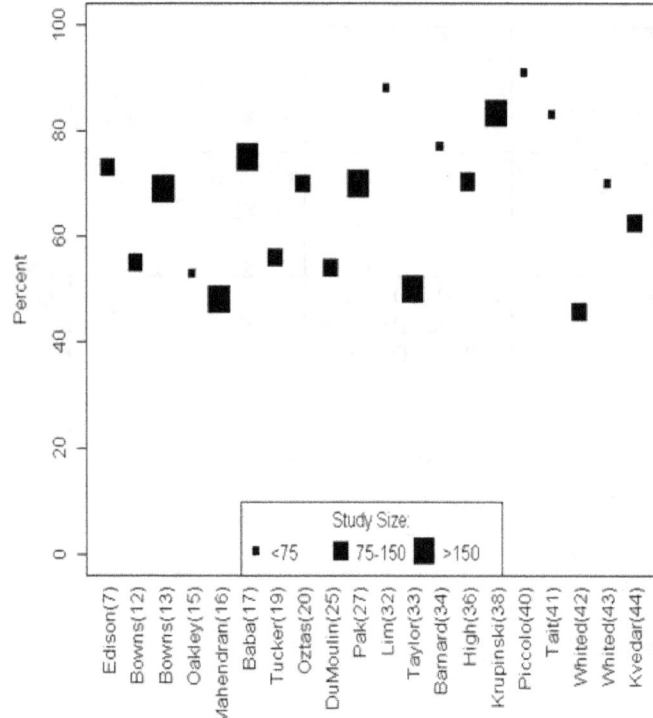

Figure 5b.

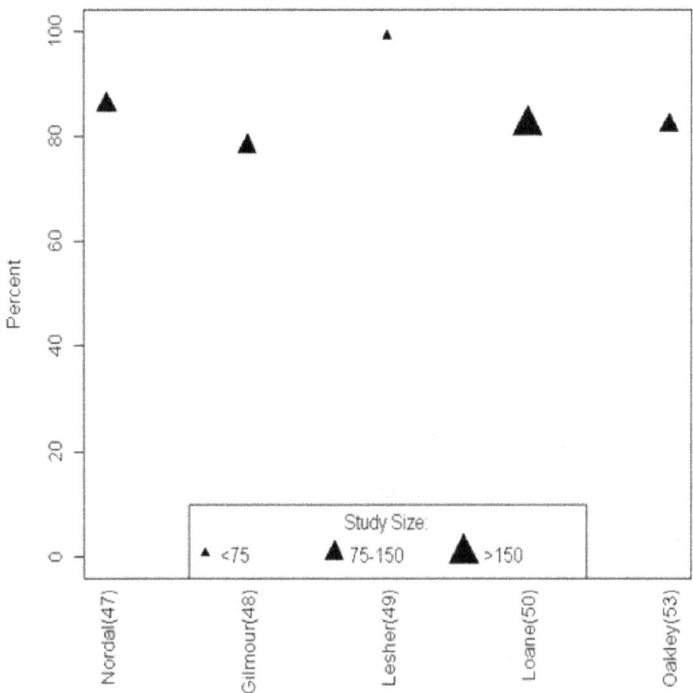

Figure 6a.

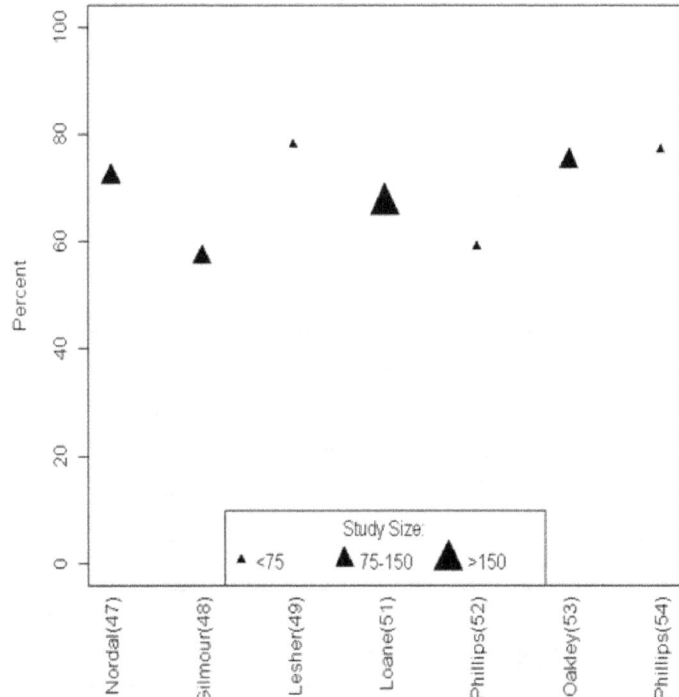

Figure 6b.

Table 5. Studies Reporting Management Accuracy using Histopathology/Lab Tests as the Gold Standard (KQ2a)

Study	TD Management Accuracy, % Correct	CD Management Accuracy, % Correct	Absolute Mean Difference, % Correct
A. Store and forward studies			
Warshaw 2009[6] VA 728 Pts 728 SL	79% (574/728)	84% (608/728)	-5%
	80% (581/728) PLD	84% (609/728) PLD	-4%
Warshaw 2009[5] VA 542 Pts 542 PSL	71% (383/542)	66% (356/542)	5%
	70% (380/542) PLD	66% (356/542) PLD	4%
	74% (401/542) CID	66% (357/542) CID	8%
Weighted mean difference for studies (range of mean differences; No. studies)	**-0.6% (-5 to 5%; 2 studies)[5,6]**		
Weighted mean difference for PLD studies (range of mean differences; No. studies)	**-0.2% (-4 to 4%; 2 studies)[5,6]**		
B. Live interactive studies			
No studies			

Table 6. Studies Reporting Management Concordance between Teledermatology and Usual Care (In-Person Dermatology) (KQ2b)

Study	Percent concordant	Kappa statistic	Sensitivity and Specificity
A. Store and forward *pigmented skin lesion* studies (n=2)			
Di Stefani 2007[9] 18 Pts 465 PSL	TD1 96% TDSC TD2 96% TDSC *Denominator: # of lesions* *For 3 Management Options (Annual follow-up, Short term follow-up, Biopsy)*	TD1 k=0.68 TD2 k=0.70	NR
Joliffe 2001[31] 611 Pts 819 PSL	80% (652/819) *Concordance for refer or not refer*	NR	Sensitivity=0.69 Specificity=0.82 *Calculated on 82% of refer or not refer*
B. Store and forward *skin lesion* studies (n=5)			
Ferrandiz 2007[10] 134 SL (73% NMSC)	NR	k=0.75 (95% CI 0.71, 0.79) *Agreement on planned surgical technique*	NR
Bowns 2006[13] 256 Pts 256 SL	61% (157/256) *Concordance for refer or not refer*	NR	NR
Mahendran 2005[16] 163 Pts 163 SL	55% (90/163)	NR	NR

Shapiro 2004[23] 49 Pts 49 SL	100% (49/49) *Concordance for biopsy vs. no biopsy*	NR	Sensitivity=1.0 (95% CI 0.87, 1.00) Specificity=1.0 (95% CI 0.85, 1.00)
Whited 1998[43] VA 12 Pts 10 SL	TD1 100% (10/10) TD2 90% (9/10) *Concordance for biopsy or no biopsy*	NR	NR
C. Store and forward *general* studies (n=7)			
Edison 2008[7] 110 Pts 110 Conditions	66% (73/110) (95% CI 58%, 75%)	k=0.62 (95% CI 0.55, 0.69)	NR
Bowns 2006[12] 92 Pts 92 Conditions	55% (51/92)	NR	NR
Oakley 2006[15] 73 Pts 109 Conditions	82% (208/252) TDSC Denominator: # of responses from up to 38 TDs and 5 CDs, including 2 plastic surgeons	NR	NR
Pak 2003[26] DoD 404 Pts 404 Conditions	76% (307/404) *Concordance for biopsy or no biopsy*	NR	NR

Whited 1999[42]
VA
129 Pts
168 Conditions *Denominators for Management Types NR*
	3 TDs
	Medical Therapy:
	   Aggregated: 71%, 75%, 80%
	   Primary: 67%, 68%, 69%
	Clinical Procedures:
	   Aggregated: 64%, 73%, 74%
	   Primary: 64%, 73%, 74%
	Diagnostic Tests:
	   Aggregated: 70%, 69%, 69%
	   Primary: 67%, 66%, 68%
		NR	NR

Lyon 1997[45] 90 Pts 90 Conditions	94% (85/90) CD=resident TD=staff	NR	NR
Zelickson 1997[46] 29 Pts 30 Conditions	90% (54/60) *Combination of 2-3 TDs*	NR	NR
D. Live interactive studies (n=4)			
Edison 2008[7] 110 Pts 110 Conditions	75% (82/110) (95% CI 66%, 83%)	k=0.71 (95% CI 0.64, 0.78)	NR
Gilmour 1998[48] 61 Pts 61 Conditions	72% (44/61)	NR	NR
Loane 1998[56] 214 Pts 252 Conditions	64% (160/252) TD also served as CD in 44% of cases	NR	NR
Phillips 1998[52] 51 Pts 107 SL	86% (92/107) *Concordance for biopsy or no biopsy*	k=0.47 *Biopsy or no biopsy*	NR

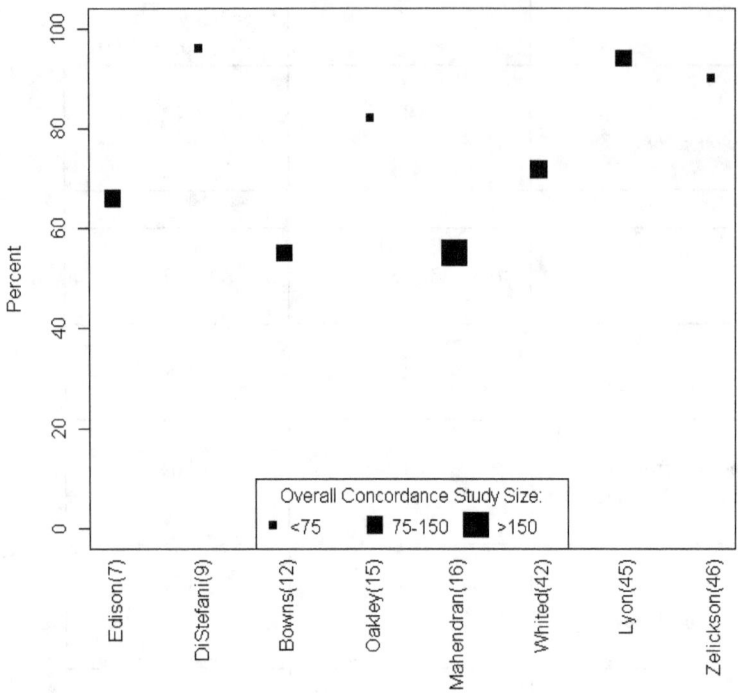

Figure 7a.

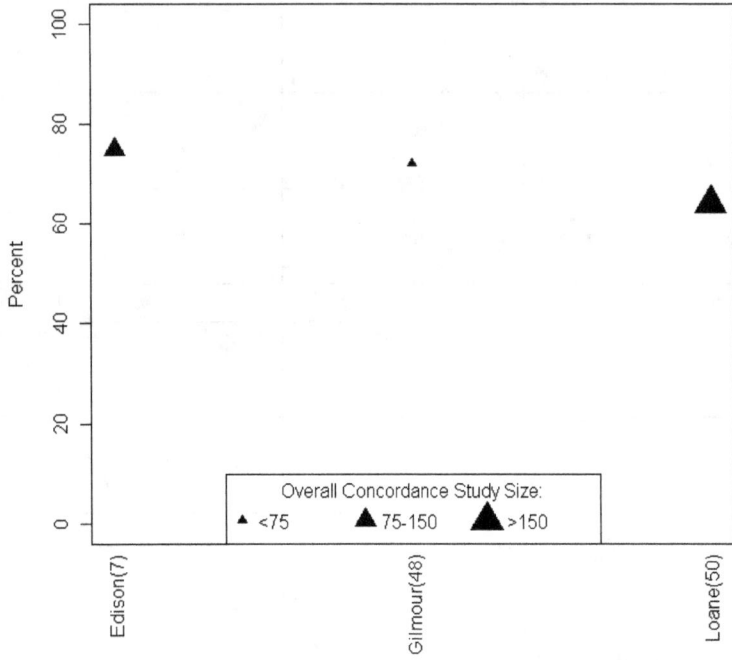

Figure 7b.

KEY QUESTION 3

How do clinical outcomes (clinical course, satisfaction, quality of life, visits avoided) of teledermatology compare to usual care (in-person dermatology) for skin conditions? (Tables 7, 8, and 9)

Clinical Outcomes: We identified three studies that reported clinical course for patients evaluated with either teledermatology or usual care (in-person dermatology) (Table 7).[57,58,59] Although two of the studies suggested that clinical course is more favorable following teledermatology, the three studies used different methods for determining clinical course and assessed clinical course at different time points.

Eminovic et al.[57] reported a notable difference in the percentage of patients improved at one month after referral in the teledermatology group (20%) compared to the usual care group (4%). The assessment was done by a dermatologist during an in-person dermatology consultation. However, it is important to note that the teledermatology group was treated during the one month period, as needed, based on the results of the teledermatology consultation while the usual care group had yet to see a dermatologist. In the Pak et al.[58] study involving DOD and veterans, the assessment was done for both groups at four months after the initial visit (either teledermatology or in-person dermatology) using photographic images. There was no significant difference in clinical course rating (improved, no change, or worse) between the two groups. Granlund et al.[59] assessed outcomes at six months using a questionnaire. The response rate was 60%. A significantly higher percentage of teledermatology patients reported that their condition had resolved (63% vs. 23%, p=0.03).

Table 7. Clinical Course Outcome for Teledermatology Studies (KQ3)

Study Country Number of Subjects for Clinical Course Outcome/Total Number of Subjects Design	Intervention	Clinical Course	
		Teledermatology	Usual Care
A. Store and forward systems studies (n=2)			
Eminovic 2009[57] Netherlands N=369 evaluable (total N=605 pts) RCT; general practitioners randomized to TD or UC Clinical outcome assessed at time of CD appointment	Teledermatology group: SAF TD followed by CD visit at 1 month Usual care group: referred for CD visit (approximately 1 month waiting time)	40/200 (20%) judged to not need CD visit because condition had improved	7/169 (4%) judged to not need CD visit because condition had improved
Pak 2007[58] United States VA and DoD N=508/698 Clinical outcome assessed by photographs (baseline compared to four months)	Teledermatology group: baseline SAF TD with repeat imaging at 4 months Usual care group: CD visit (baseline) with imaging for outcome assessment only; repeat imaging at 4 months	64% improved 33% no change 4% worse n=272	65% improved 32% no change 3% worse n=236 (p=0.57)
B. Live interactive studies (n=1)			
Granlund 2003[59] Finland N=29/48 Non-randomized; same dermatologist for TD and UC Clinical outcome assessed via questionnaire at six months (29 of 48 pts responded)	Patients from first clinic had TD consultation Patients from second clinic had CD consultation Both groups: follow-up as needed after initial consultation	63% "still suffer from disease" 63% "resolved" n=16	85% "still suffer from disease" 23% "resolved" n=13 (p=0.03)

Patient Satisfaction: Seven SAF and four LI studies reported patient satisfaction (Table 8). Assessment tools ranged from a single question to surveys with over 50 items. As a result of the wide discrepancy in assessments used, we focused our report on overall satisfaction measures rather than satisfaction with specific elements of teledermatology or usual care (in-person dermatology).

SAF Studies: In the four SAF studies that included both teledermatology and usual care groups, satisfaction ratings were comparable with a mean satisfaction rating of 3.8 out of 5,[57] or greater than 75% of patients reporting satisfaction with both teledermatology and usual care.[12,18,60] In the three studies with no comparison group, teledermatology was rated as "excellent" or "good" by 42% of the patients;[61] 93% reported they were "happy" with teledermatology;[62,63] and at 4 to 6 weeks after teledermatology, 64% reported they were satisfied.[64] Three of the studies included VA or DoD populations.[60,61,64]

LI Studies: Four LI studies reported patient satisfaction. In the one study that included teledermatology and usual care groups (non-randomized), a significantly greater number of patients (96% vs. 83%, p=0.03) reported they were satisfied with teledermatology than with usual care.[59] The median satisfaction rating (on a scale of 0 to 10) was also higher for the teledermatology group (9.6 vs. 9.0, p=0.03). Of the three studies without a comparison group, the reported satisfaction ratings were 44%,[47] 88%,[65] and 92%.[66] Only one of these studies was completed in the United States.[65]

Overall: Of the five studies that included both teledermatology (either SAF or LI) and usual care groups, patients expressed comparable levels of satisfaction in three of the studies (all of which were randomized, controlled trials; one included a veteran population).[12,57,60] One non-randomized study reported greater satisfaction with teledermatology.[59] One repeated measures study reported greater satisfaction with usual care, however, the usual care patients in that study had already been seen via SAF teledermatology.[18] Response rates for the satisfaction assessments ranged from 58% to 100%.

Patient Preference: Four SAF and eight LI studies reported patient preference (Table 8). A total of four of these studies (2 SAF, 2 LI) were conducted in the United States.

SAF Studies: With the exception of one study that reported that 76% of patients preferred teledermatology over waiting for a usual care appointment,[12] preferences for teledermatology or usual care were similar. In one VA study, 42% preferred teledermatology over usual care while 37% preferred usual care over teledermatology.[60] A study from the United Kingdom reported that 40% preferred usual care over teledermatology with 68% responded that teledermatology was "as good as" usual care.[62,63] A DoD-based study reported that 42% preferred teledermatology and 38% preferred usual care when asked 4 to 6 weeks after their initial appointment.[64]

LI Studies: In one study, patients experienced both SAF and LI sessions. Although 85% "accepted" SAF teledermatology, 82% of those patients felt that the LI session was also needed.[17] Reported preferences for teledermatology ranged from 69%[65] to 38%.[47,48] Reported preferences for usual care ranged from 28%[47] to 43%.[67] In two studies, approximately one-third of the patients surveyed expressed no preference.[47,53] In two studies, teledermatology was rated "as good as" usual care by 54%[53] and 66%[67] of patients.

Overall: Preference for teledermatology ranged from 38% to 86%. One study reported slightly higher satisfaction with usual care but 76% of the patients preferred teledermatology over waiting to see a dermatologist.[12] A VA study reported that patients were more likely to respond "strongly agree" to statements about satisfaction with usual care and more likely to respond "agree" to statements about satisfaction with teledermatology yet "most" patients preferred a teledermatology appointment rather than driving 2 hours to see a dermatologist.[51] It appears that other factors, such as waiting time for a in-person dermatology appointment and the need to travel long distances (involving both expense and time off from work), influence patient preference for usual care or teledermatology.

Table 8. Patient Satisfaction and Patient Preference for Teledermatology Studies (KQ3)

Study Country Satisfaction Assessment Number of Patients for this Outcome Preference	Patient Satisfaction		Preference
	Teledermatology	Usual Care	
A. Store and forward systems studies (n=7)			
Eminovic 2009[57] Netherlands RCT - GPs randomized to TD or UC 20/43 items from short-form Patient Satisfaction Questionnaire III (mean score, 5 point scale - 5 indicating greatest satisfaction) N=350/605 (57.8% response rate)	3.8 n=191	3.8 n=159	NR
Bowns 2006[12] United Kingdom RCT 51 items from Patient Satisfaction Questionnaire III plus 9 items specific to SAF N=147/208 (70.7% response rate)	satisfied overall: 84% n=80	satisfied overall: 87% n=67 (p=0.59)	preferred TD over waiting for UC: 76%
Moreno-Ramirez 2005[18] Spain, Pigmented Lesions Repeated measure design Question "Are you satisfied with this way of being attended by a specialist?" N=219 TD; 108/219 "selected" for additional UC	very satisfied: 86% n=219	very satisfied: 98% n=108 (all had TD before UC)	NR
Whited 2004[60] United States; Durham, NC VAMC RCT Telephone Survey UC: Visit-Specific Satisfaction Questionnaire TD: Related questions plus specific TD items BOTH: 5 point scale (Excellent to Poor) N=194/275 (70.5% response rate)	excellent or very good: 79% n=101	excellent or very good: 78% n=93	preferred TD over UC: 42% preferred UC over TD: 37%

Weinstock 2001[61]
United States; Togus, Maine VAMC
TD Cohort
Telephone Survey (10 questions)
    5 point scale (Excellent to Poor)
    Mean 14 months after TD (range 2.5-30.5)
N=100/148 (67.6% response rate) randomly selected
    from 1030 consults
	excellent or good:
	42%
	
	ability of TD to treat skin disease:
	    good/excellent 41%
	      fair/poor 46%
		no comparison group	NR

Williams 2001[62,63] United Kingdom TD Cohort Survey of 15 items developed for SAF TD 5 point scale (strongly disagree to strongly agree) N=123/141 (87.2% response rate)	"happy" with TD: 93%	no comparison group	prefer UC to TD: 40% believed TD as good as UC: 68%

Pak 1999[64]
United States, DoD
TD Cohort
Survey (details NR) at baseline and 4-6 weeks
N=77/100 (baseline; 77% response rate)
N= 55/100 (4-6 week; 55% response rate)
	baseline:
	    satisfied with TD:
	    "most"
	
	4-6 weeks:
	    satisfied with TD:
	64%
		no comparison group	at 4-6 weeks:
			    prefer UC: 38%
			    prefer TD to waiting for
			      UC: 42%

B. Live interactive studies (n=9)			

Granlund 2003[59]
Finland
Open, non-randomized TD vs. UC
Survey of 5 questions:
    Completed after encounter and 6 months
    5 point scale (very good to very bad)
Linear analog scale of 0 to 10
    Completed after encounter and 6 months
N=48 immediately after encounter
N=29 at 6 months
	satisfied with TD:
	96%
	    n=23
	
	Linear analog scale:
	    Median=9.6 after consultation
	    Mean=7.4 at 6 months
	    n=16
		satisfied with UC: 83%
		n=25 (p=0.03)
		
		Linear analog scale:
		    Median=9.0 after consultation
		    (p=0.03)
		    Mean=6.6 at 6 months
		    (p>0.05)
		    n=13
			NR

Baba 2005[17]
Turkey
Combined SAF + LI Cohort
Questions:
    1) Acceptance of TD or UC
    2) Need for LI in addition to SAF
N=228
	overall satisfaction NR	no comparison group	would accept TD:
			85% (of these, 82% felt LI+SAF was needed rather than just SAF)

Hicks 2003[65]
United States
TD Cohort
Survey of 8 questions:
    Completed after each visit, ≥1 survey per pt
    7-point scale (very unsatisfied to very satisfied)
N=321 TD pts
	very satisfied or satisfied: 88%
	n=258
		no comparison group	felt TD much better/better than UC: 69%
			n=255

Nordal 2001[47]
Norway
Repeated measures design
Survey of 9 items:
    4 point scale (very satisfied to unsatisfied)
N=116/121 (95.9% response rate)
	very satisfied with TD: 44%
	
	unsatisfied with TD: 10%
		no comparison group	for a future dermatology consult:
			    prefer TD: 38%
			    prefer UC: 28%
			    indifferent: 34%
			general preference:
			    prefer TD: 18%
			    prefer CD: 16%
			    indifferent: 66%

Lamminen 2000[66] Finland TD Cohort Survey (details NR) N=25	TD "excellent or good": 92%	no comparison group	NR
Gilmour 1998[48] United Kingdom Repeated measures design Survey of 16 items: 5 point scale (strongly disagree to strongly agree) N=122/126 (96.8% response)	overall satisfaction NR	no comparison group	prefer TD: 38% prefer UC: 42% TD as good as UC: 43%
Lowitt 1998[51] United States, Baltimore VAMC Repeated measures design Survey of 7 items: 4 point scale (strongly disagree to strongly agree) N=124/139 (89.2% response rate)	overall satisfaction NR	overall satisfaction NR more "strongly agree" responses for UC vs. more "agree" responses for TD (p=0.001)	"most" prefer TD close to home rather than UC 2 hours away
Loane 1998[67] Northern Ireland Repeated measures design Survey of 15 items: 5 point scale (strongly disagree to strongly agree) N=292/334 (87.4% response rate)	overall satisfaction NR	overall satisfaction NR	prefer TD: 41% prefer UC: 43% TD as good as UC: 66%
Oakley 1997[53] New Zealand Repeated measures design Survey (details NR): 5 point scale (strongly disagree to strongly agree) N=98/104 (94.2% response rate)	overall satisfaction NR	overall satisfaction NR	TD as good as UC: 54% undecided: 31%

<u>Time to Treatment:</u> Four SAF studies and no LI studies addressed the question of time to treatment (Table 9). One study included both time to treatment and time to teledermatology results; one additional study included only time to teledermatology results.

In all four studies, the time to treatment was shorter for patients who were initially seen by teledermatology. Time from general practitioner consult to dermatology clinic (or opinion) was significantly shorter for teledermatology patients compared to usual care patients in the three studies that reported this outcome[11,12,68] with the difference ranging from 44 days to 76.3 days (all p<0.001). Time to biopsy was 19 days shorter (p=0.03).[68] Time to surgery or definitive intervention was significantly shorter in the three studies that reported this outcome.[10,68,69] The difference ranged from 21 to 86 days (all p<0.01). Two of these studies[68,69] were conducted at VA medical centers. It is important to note that although times to treatment experienced by teledermatology patients in the VA studies were shorter than those for usual care patients, the reported times are not reflective of current VA practices; all veterans now are scheduled within 30 days. Two studies reported time to teledermatology results. Mean times were 61.1 hours[11] and 44 hours.[18]

Clinic Dermatology Visits Avoided: The number of in-person dermatology visits avoided was reported in 11 SAF and 3 LI studies (Table 9). Two SAF studies reported the number of dermatology visits required. Teledermatology patients required a mean of 0.98 visits in one study[68] and 1 visit in another study.[10] In the same two studies, usual care patients required a mean of 1.13 or at least 2 visits, respectively.

Two SAF studies reported the percentage of patients who did not require a dermatology clinic visit ("preventable" visits) following teledermatology compared to usual care patients. The differences between groups were 20.7% (39% teledermatology vs. 18.3% usual care)[57] and 28% (66% teledermatology vs. 38% usual care).[12] Two live interactive studies reported a similar outcome with a difference of 14% (44% teledermatology vs. 30% usual care) in one study[70] and a difference favoring usual care of 1% (54% teledermatology vs. 55% usual care).[71]

Seven additional SAF studies and one additional LI study reported visits avoided with no comparison group. The percentage of visits avoided ranged from 12.8% to 72%.[11,16,18,33,64,66,69,72] The study that reported 12.8% clinic dermatology visits avoided also reported that 33.1% required clinic dermatology surgery.[16]

Conclusions: There was insufficient evidence to conclude whether teledermatology had an effect on clinical course, although a VA/DoD study with over 500 patients reported comparable outcomes. Patient overall satisfaction with and preference for teledermatology or usual care were comparable in VA/DoD and other studies. Patients noted waiting time for an appointment and travel time/distance as factors when considering preference. Time to treatment was significantly shorter and clinic dermatology visits can be avoided when patients have an initial teledermatology visit.

Table 9. Time to Treatment and Clinic Dermatology Visits Avoided for Teledermatology Studies (KQ3)

Study	Time to Treatment (Average)	CD Visits Avoided*
A. Store and forward systems studies (n=11)		
Eminovic 2009[57] Netherlands Cluster RCT N=369/605	NR	CD visits "preventable" for: TD 39.0% (N=200) UC 18.3% (N=169) Difference 20.7% (95% CI 8.5, 32.9)
Hsiao 2008[68] United States Retrospective review of veterans treated for skin cancer N=149/169 46% UC, 54% TD	Consult to (days): Opinion (TD or CD): TD 4 vs. UC 48 (p<0.001) Biopsy: TD 38 vs. UC 57 (p=0.034) Surgery: TD 104 vs. UC 125 (p=0.006)	Mean number of CD visits: TD 0.98 vs. UC 1.13 (p=0.02) NOTE: 14% of TD did not require any CD visits prior to surgery; all UC required ≥1 visit
Ferrandiz 2007[10] Spain Pilot study of SL needing regular surgical excision N=226 (134 TD compared to random sample of 92 UC	Consult to surgery (days): TD 26.1 vs. UC 60.6 (p<0.001)	TD: 1 CD visit needed UC: ≥ 2 CD visits needed Difference: ≥ 1 visit
Moreno-Ramirez 2007[11] Spain Repeated Measure, Historical Control N=2539 (2009 TD compared to 530 UC	Consult to CD clinic (days): TD 12.3 vs. UC 88.6 (p<0.001) Time for TD results 61.1 hrs NOTE: N unclear for this outcome	51.2% (n=1029) of TD did not need CD visit
Bowns 2006[12] United Kingdom RCT N=165/208	Consult to opinion (days): TD 13 (n=85) vs. UC 67 (n=72) p<0.0001	No follow-up visits needed: TD 66% vs. UC 38% (p=0.0003)
Knol 2006[72] Netherlands N=306 intent to refer consultations and 505 TD No comparison group	NR	53.3% (n=163) did not need CD
Mahendran 2005[16] United Kingdom Repeated Measure N=163	NR	12.8% (n=21) did not need CD (reassurance only) 33.1% (n=54) did not need CD consult visit but did need CD surgery
Moreno-Ramirez 2005[18] Spain Cohort, PSL N=219	Time for TD results 44 hrs	51% (n=111) did not need CD
Whited 2002[69] United States RCT of Veterans N=275 (TD=135, UC=127)	Consult to definitive intervention (days, median): Intent to Treat: TD 41 vs. UC 127 p=0.0001 Actual Visit: TD 50 vs. UC 137.5 p=0.0027	18.5% of TD did not need CD
Taylor 2001[33] United Kingdom TD Reliability Study N=188/194	NR	31% of TD did not need CD (based on 376 assessments, 188 cases X 2 consultants) NOTE: CD diagnosis differed from TD diagnosis in 14% of these 188 cases

Pak 1999[64] United States Department of Defense Cohort, no comparison group N=100	NR		45% did not need CD
B. Live interactive studies (n=3)			
Loane 2001[70] United Kingdom RCT TD vs. UC N=274 (126 TD, 148 UC)	NR		44% of TD and 30% of UC did not need follow-up visit
Wooton 2000[71] United Kingdom RCT TD vs. UC N=204 (102 TD, 102 UC)	NR		54% of TD and 55% of UC did not need follow-up visit
Lamminen 2000[66] Finland Cohort, TD N=25	NR		72% did not need follow-up visit

*Does not include TD visit(s). Number of CD visits avoided

KEY QUESTION 4

How does the cost of teledermatology compare to usual care (in-person dermatology)? (Table 10)

Cost data were reported in three studies involving SAF teledermatology, six studies of LI teledermatology, and one study that included both SAF and LI teledermatology (Table 10). Due to differences in factors included in cost assessments and the various perspectives (societal, health service, or patient), it was difficult to summarize these findings.

SAF Studies: Whited et al.[73] used a micro-costing approach with a VA perspective and found that teledermatology was cost-effective but not cost-saving for decreasing time to initial definitive dermatologic care. It was assumed that VA centers had both on-site primary care and dermatology clinics. Definitive care was achieved in 50 days using teledermatology compared to 138 days with usual care. The long-duration to achieve definitive dermatologic care, particularly for the usual care population, is no longer consistent with current VA practice (appointments within 30 days) and may result in an overly favorable estimate of teledermatology. Pak et al.,[74] based on a DoD population, reported cost savings of $32 per patient if lost productivity was considered. Moreno-Ramirez et al.[75] reported that teledermatology was cost-effective for patients referred to a skin cancer clinic.

SAF and LI Study: A comparison of SAF and LI teledermatology found store and forward to be less expensive but less efficient clinically than live interactive teledermatology.[80] This analysis considered the educational benefit to general practitioners obtained during the live interactive sessions.

LI Studies: Six studies assessed LI versus usual care including two studies conducted in the United States. Studies had marked differences in design and settings. Most indicated that teledermatology either cost less or was cost efficient compared to usual care, particularly if patients had to travel long distances or certain criteria were met for referral volume and costs.

<u>Conclusions:</u> Cost studies were limited by variations in parameters included and perspectives chosen for the analyses. The majority of studies (including both SAF and LI technologies) found teledermatology to be cost effective if certain critical assumptions were met; the most important included patient travel distance, teledermatology volume, and costs of usual care.

Table 10. Teledermatology Studies Reporting Cost Outcomes (KQ4)

Author/Year/Country Funding Design	Participants Age, race, gender Skin Conditions	Sites Providers Assumptions	Cost Outcomes/Utilization Outcomes (US$, except as noted)
Store and Forward vs. Usual Care (N=3)			
Whited 2003[73] U.S. Veterans VA HSR&D RCT TD vs. UC	N=275 (135 TD, 140 UC) age: NR race: NR gender: NR Conditions: NR	On-site primary care clinic and on-site dermatology clinic Providers: primarily dermatology residents Micro-costing approach, VA perspective	-Average cost ($) per pt (base-case): TD: 36.40 UC: 21.40 Incremental cost per pt: 15.00 (sensitivity analysis range: 10.50 to 15.00) -Median time to initial definitive intervention: TD: 50.0 days UC: 137.5 days Incremental effectiveness: 87.5 days Incremental cost-effectiveness ratio for TD: $0.17 per pt per day (sensitivity analysis range: $0.12 to $0.17) Conclusion: TD not cost-saving but was cost-effective for decreasing time to initial definitive dermatological care
Pak 2009[74] U.S. Army Personnel U.S. Army Telemedicine and Advanced Technology Research Center RCT TD vs. UC	N=698 (351 TD, 347 UC) age: NR race: NR gender: NR Conditions: NR	Military primary care and dermatology clinics Providers: NR Cost-minimization, DoD perspective	-Costs ($, average per pt) TD UC Total Direct 103,043 (294) 98,365 (283) Lost Productivity 16,359 (47) 30,768 (89) Total Cost 119,402 (340) 129,133 (372) Conclusion: TD cost-saving, if lost productivity is considered
Moreno-Ramirez 2009[75] Spain Instituto Carlos III Non-randomized comparison of consecutive TD and UC pts	N=4018 (2009 TD, 2009 UC) age: NR race: NR gender: NR Conditions: suspected skin cancer	12 primary care clinics/ 1 central skin cancer clinic Providers: NR Societal perspective	-Waiting interval for skin cancer clinic: TD: 12.3 days UC: 88.6 days Incremental effectiveness 76.3 days -Unit cost ($) per pt: TD: 119.67 UC: 194.06 (p<0.005) Incremental cost savings of TD $74.39 -Cost-effectiveness: $0.98 saved per waiting day avoided by TD Conclusion: SAF TD is cost-effective for referrals to skin cancer clinic

Store and Forward vs. Live Interactive (N=1)

Loane†
2000[80]
United Kingdom
 	
NHS R&D, Southern Health and Social Services Board, Glaxo, Steifel
 	
Repeated measure – both SAF and LI TD
 	
Anonymous economic questionnaire after LI consultation
	N=96 /102 randomized to TD (see Wootton 2000)
	
	age: mean=38.9 years
	race: NR
	gender: 47% male
	
	Conditions: Most common - eczema, psoriasis, acne, and tumors
		4 primary care centers (2 rural, 2 urban) and 2 dermatology centers
		
		Providers: 2 dermatologists (1 for SAF and 1 for LI)
			-Dermatologist consultation time (mean):
			 SAF: 1.6 min LI: 15.7 min
			-Total pt time (wait, consult, travel) (mean):
			 SAF: 41.5 min LI: 52.2 min
			-Variable costs per pt
			                    SAF LI
			 Dermatologist £4.00 £39.25
			 GP £9.50 £29.83
			 Pt time off work £4.76 £5.99
			 Pt travel (all local) £1.89 £1.89
			    Total £20.15 £76.96
			-Fixed costs SAF: £6.75 LI: £124.92
			-Savings with LI (20% non-referral savings): £9.74
			-Benefits with LI (GP training): £60.04
			-Net societal costs SAF: £29.90 LI: £132.10
			
			Conclusion: SAF cheaper, but less clinically efficient, than LI

Live Interactive vs. Usual Care (N=6)

Burgiss 1997[76] U.S. Funding: NR Before and after TD comparison	N=87 (119 visits) age: NR race: NR gender: NR Conditions: dermatitis, infectious, acneiform, papulosquamous, tumors	2 rural primary care centers and university dermatology clinic Providers: 1 dermatologist	-Total Costs $ (per Pt) Primary care* TD Provider 8,848 (102) 5,236 (60) Diagnostic evaluation 9,367 (108) 3,031 (35) Medication 7,388 (85) 3,969 (46) Total 25,603 (294) 12,236 (141) *cost of care for pt prior to TD consultation Conclusion: TD can decrease costs of dermatological care
Wootton† 2000[71] United Kingdom UK Multicentre Teledermatology Trial NHS R&D; Southern Health and Social Service Board, Glaxo, Steifel RCT TD vs. UC Anonymous economic questionnaire after TD consultation	N=169/204 (102 TD, 102 UC) age: mean=38.6 yrs race: NR gender: 42% male Conditions: NR	4 primary care centers (2 rural, 2 urban) and 2 dermatology centers Providers: NR	-Costs per Pt TD UC Variable costs £76.96 £48.73 Fixed costs £124.92 £0.00 Savings £9.74 £0.00 Benefits £60.04 £0.00 Net societal cost £132.10 £48.73 Conclusion: TD not cost-effective in setting evaluated (average distance to dermatology clinic 26km); TD would be cost-effective if distance >78km

Study	Population	Costs	Setting
Loane 2001[77] New Zealand New Zealand Ministry of Health and Health Informatics Foundation, V-Tel, B&H Ltd, Digital Equipment Corporation, Leo RCT TD vs. UC Patient questionnaire	N=203 (109 TD, 94 UC) age: mean=41 yrs (14% minors/in school) race: NR gender: 48% male Conditions: NR	-Costs ($): TD UC Fixed Costs 7974.05 0.00 Variable Costs 7481.45 13,536.60 Total 15,455.50 13,536.60 Unit Cost 125.65 127.71 Conclusion: From societal perspective, TD more cost-efficient than UC	2 rural primary care centers and 1 dermatology department Providers: NR Societal perspective Conditions: NR

Bergmo 2000[78]
Norway
 	
Funding: NR
 	
Case Series comparison of TD to 3 alternatives:
1. combination of pt travel and visiting dermatologist
2. pt travel to central dermatologist
3. hiring local dermatologist
	N=375 TD pts (actual workload for 1 yr)
	
	age: NR
	race: NR
	gender: NR
	
	Conditions: NR
		-Fixed Costs ($)
		  TD: 43,866.35 Pt Travel/Visiting: 35,052.60
		  Pt Travel: 0 Local Dermatologist: 105,452.60
		-Variable Costs ($) per Pt
		  TD: 21.12 Pt Travel/Visiting: 66.33 for 1st 240 pts*
		  Pt Travel: 479.60 Local Dermatologist: 0
		*Maximum workload for visiting dermatologist - 240 pts; remaining pts travel to clinic at cost of $339.90 per pt
		
		Conclusion: TD was less costly than the three alternatives if >195 pts per year
			1 primary care clinic and 1 central dermatology clinic
			
			Providers: NR
			
			Assumed health outcomes for TD = UC
			
			Societal and health-care sector perspective

Loane† 2001[70]
UK
 	
Funding :NR
 	
RCT TD vs. UC
 	
Patient questionnaire after each visit
	N=274 pts (126 TD, 148 UC)
	254/413 (62%) questionnaires completed
	
	age: mean=39.7 years
	race: NR
	gender: 44% male
	
	TD pts: 61% urban, 39% rural
	UC pts: 71% urban, 29% rural
	
	Conditions: NR
		-Total Costs/Benefits($):
		              Urban Rural
		             TD UC TD UC
		Variable 7025 7226 4747 3062
		Fixed 10527 0 8605 0
		Total 17552 7226 13352 3062
		Savings 1084 0 459 0
		Societal* 16468 7226 12893 3062
		Marginal** 77 69 88 71
		Unit*** 214 69 263 71
		*(Fixed+Variable)-(Savings)
		**(Variable-Savings)/(#Pts)
		***(Societal)/(#Pts)
		
		Conclusion: Overall, total costs higher for TD than UC
		Sensitivity analysis found that for rural areas, TD costs < UC
			1 urban and 1 rural primary care clinic and 1 dermatology department
			
			Providers: General practitioners and dermatologists
			
			Health service and pt perspectives

Armstrong 2007[79] U.S. Funding: NR Non-randomized comparison of TD and UC visits	N=451 TD visits (301 new, 150 follow-up) and 47,434 UC visits age: NR race: NR gender: NR Conditions: Top 5 conditions: actinic keratosis, eczema, acne, benign neo-plasm, viral infection	1 Primary care center and 1 dermatology clinic Providers: 1 nurse prac-titioner (trained in der-matologic procedures); 1 dermatologist Provider perspective; cost-minimization	-Costs ($) per hour		
				TD	UC
			TD equipment	4.75	0.00
			Facility and personnel	143.88	193.04
			Physician compensation	125.00	153.00
			Total	273.63	346.04
			Conclusion: Hourly costs higher for UC than TD One-way Sensitivity Analyses found TD = UC costs if: a. technology cost $44/hr b. physician compensation was $197/hr c. clinic space cost was $57/hr (rather than $12.50-TD and $100-UC) Reimbursement for TD: per visit=$122, per hour=$487		

†UK Multicentre Teledermatology Trial

1. Post-operative wound care, and chronic dermatitis.

KEY QUESTION 5

What are the key structural and process elements associated with successful implementation of teledermatology and what are the barriers? (Table 11)

As summarized above, most research in teledermatology has focused on the accuracy and reliability to diagnose and manage skin conditions in a research setting. However, lessons learned from mature, functioning teledermatology systems include "…that the successful implementation of teledermatology as a routine service requires understanding of and paying great attention to the interplay between social and technical aspects of teledermatology."[81] Finch and colleagues conducted a longitudinal qualitative study based on in-depth semi-structured interviews of dermatologists, nurses, administrators, patient advocates, primary care providers and technologists in 12 teledermatology services in the UK and concluded that "the original… vision of how teledermatology would be utilized, as a technological fix for long waiting lists and consultant shortages, failed to be realized."[82]

Several publications have described key elements for successful implementation of teledermatology.[83,84,85,86,87,88,89] We summarized these recommendations in Table 11. We attempted to categorize success facilitators using the definitions of Greenhalgh et al.[3] We categorized implementation barriers according to administrative, clinical, patient and technical factors. We emphasized factors likely to play a role in VA specific settings. Detailed information on specific equipment, training in photography, and computerized medical record applications are beyond the scope of this review and are available on the World Wide Web.[90,91,92] Because store and forward is the method used almost exclusively for dermatology in the VA system (informal survey December, 2009), we focused on this form of teledermatology in this section. Readers interested in lessons learned from live interactive teledermatology programs are referred to Oakley et al.[1] The following summary of key elements of facilitators and barriers to implementation are based on a review of the literature and the authors' experience with teledermatology within the VA.

<u>Evaluate the Implementation Setting:</u>

Prior to implementing a teledermatology program, a thorough evaluation of organizational issues for the specific VA setting is critical. Most Veterans Integrated Service Networks (VISNs) have at least one larger medical center with dermatology services whereas smaller VAMCs and Community Based Outpatient Clinics (CBOCs) usually do not have on-site dermatology services. There are three likely scenarios for implementing teledermatology in a VA setting:

Intrasite Service: Teledermatology services for a site which already has an onsite VA dermatology service. The main purpose of this type of service is usually triaging dermatology consults.

Intersite Service: Teledermatology services for a site which has no onsite VA dermatology services but a VA with a dermatology clinic is within reasonable driving distance.

New Service: Teledermatology services for a site which has no VA dermatology services. In this scenario, dermatology services are usually either provided by community dermatologists (fee basis or contract), by other VA specialties (surgery, ophthalmology, plastics, infectious diseases, etc), or by primary care without specialty support.

Define Objectives:

The objectives for these three VA scenarios may be very different. As described by Pak,[83] common objectives of teledermatology programs include: to improve access to dermatology, to optimize dermatology resources, to reduce dermatology costs, and/or to improve quality of health care (including educating primary care physicians). Identifying specific objectives will help determine the type of teledermatology service best suited for the program's goals. Because new systems require significant effort, it is crucial that key players (dermatologists, primary care providers, and administrators) perceive that the benefits outweigh the effort and commitment to learning a new system. In the framework of Rogers[2] this would be considered determining the relative advantage of teledermatology versus existing services.

Understand Organizational Issues:

Understanding how the VISN or specific medical center delivers dermatological care is important. This is consistent with the Greenhalgh et al.[3] recommendation that implementation of teledermatology must be compatible with medical center's existing values, behaviors and past experiences. Lessons learned from teledermatology in the United Kingdom include that teledermatology is "not a quick nor simple fix for long waiting times in dermatology."[82] Revenue models for Intrasite and Intersite situations are relatively simple as the main dermatology service already provides dermatology care. In these situations, the main goal is often to decrease waiting times and eliminate unnecessary visits to the dermatology clinic; physician workload generally remains stable for dermatology but may increase for primary care. For the New Service scenario, workload for both the dermatology hub site and remote primary care site increase. In this situation, fee basis/consultation costs for the remote site generally decrease; if the two sites have different operating budgets, there will need to be some type of transfer of funds to support the extra workload by the dermatology service. It is also important to realize that not all skin conditions are treatable via teledermatology, so some fee basis/consultation by the referring site to community dermatologists will continue in the New Service scenario and therefore, it is unlikely that these costs will be completely eliminated.

Evaluate and Provide Required Resources:

It is important to evaluate the resources (primary care, dermatology, and other specialty resources) at each site. For the Intrasite and Intersite situations, resources are usually a minor concern because any services not available in primary care are usually available in dermatology, which is either on site (Intrasite) or within driving distance (Intersite). There may be some simple resources needed in primary care (e.g., liquid nitrogen for treatment of warts and actinic keratoses) that will enhance management of common skin conditions in primary care without requiring a dermatology visit. If these additional resources are not created, teledermatology will simply function as a triage tool, eliminating only consultations for straightforward benign growths or treatment for simple skin rashes.[73] For the New Service scenario and the Intersite scenario, additional manpower will be needed for follow-up of teledermatology recommendations at the referring site. Often this is a primary care physician, physician assistant, or nurse practitioner who serves as a "local dermatology champion," someone who is willing to perform skin biopsies, microscopic examinations for fungus, bacteria and scabies, and other relatively minor procedures. If this creates extra workload for that individual, it is important that this be recognized, and if needed, adjustments made to their schedule. Because approximately 50% of VA dermatology visits are related to skin neoplasms, it is important to identify surgical specialties at the referring site for excisions of biopsy-proven skin cancers (e.g., ophthalmology, plastics, general surgery, ear/nose/throat). A key component is whether the implementation scenarios developed are of relatively low complexity and easy to understand and use for both the dermatology and the referring primary care services. In an informal survey of VA dermatology service chiefs in December 2009, three sites volunteered information regarding reasons why they discontinued providing teledermatology services which included that teledermatology: was an ineffective use of physician time, resulted in suboptimal images, and that most patients ultimately needed to come to the dermatology clinic (unpublished).

Conduct Cost Analysis and Assess Alternatives to Teledermatology

One of the most common mistakes in planning teledermatology programs is to focus primarily on the cost of teledermatology equipment. Store and forward teledermatology equipment generally consists of an off-the-shelf, moderate quality digital camera. Personnel, not equipment costs, are the most important costs in a teledermatology program and all alternatives to teledermatology should be explored. In the New Service scenario, the major alternative is outsourcing (fee basis, consultation). Other common options include hiring a part-time dermatologist or a physician extender with dermatology training. Cost comparisons of teledermatology with these alternatives should include evaluation of the number of consults, number of dermatology visits typically required per patient, average cost per consultation, and the types of services typically provided by community dermatologists. For example, if the major services provided by community dermatologists are procedures, teledermatology is unlikely to yield cost savings because these procedures cannot be performed remotely unless a VA provider is hired or trained to perform these procedures.

Prepare a Business Model

The business model needs to incorporate support at the remote site for both obtaining and uploading photographs and dermatologic-specific medical history and for follow-up of teledermatology recommendations. This "teledermatology technician" is often a nurse practitioner, physician assistant, nurse, or other medical personnel. While one study found that it took an average of 12 minutes for a primary care physician to take pictures, upload the images, and subsequently implement advice,[93] for consistency of photo quality and efficiency of physician time, we do not advocate that primary care physicians function as imagers and/or technicians. Collins and colleagues[94] collected data from 36 general practitioners (who were responsible for obtaining photographs and uploading information) participating in a randomized controlled trial of SAF teledermatology in the United Kingdom; 47% stated that they were not satisfied with teledermatology (21% were satisfied and 32% were unsure) and 50% identified increased workload as a key problem. In his review of teledermatology in the military, Pak stated that "teledermatology has not been embraced by primary care providers because it requires additional resources at the referring site (although less total resources for the higher organization). Most clinics were short on personnel and primary care providers did not have time to take photos."[85] Implementation is more likely to succeed if the teledermatology technician is not the referring provider and has flexible duties so that he/she is available to perform teledermatology services when needed so that the patient does not have to return for imaging. Alternatively, patients can be scheduled at a later time into a teledermatology clinic at the remote site for imaging by the teledermatology technician.

A process for follow-up of teledermatology patients is also critical. In some situations, the teledermatology technician also serves as a coordinator, notifying patients of teledermatology recommendations, coordinating medication recommendations, suggested procedures and appropriate follow-up visits. In all three scenarios (Intersite, Intrasite, and New Service), teledermatology involves a shift from a dermatology referral model to a co-managed/consult model and more workload for primary care providers. Unless support for this increased workload is provided, the system is likely to fail.

Obtain Organizational Support

It is important to obtain support from key opinion leaders at both the referring site and the dermatology site. Medical center leadership, primary care, surgical subspecialties, dermatology, and pharmacy are important. If the referring site does not perceive a need for teledermatology, there will be minimal incentive to allocate space and resources. For the Intersite and New Service scenarios, the remote pharmacy may need to stock additional dermatology-specific medications and create quick pharmacy orders in the VA Computerized Patient Record System (CPRS). "Marketing" teledermatology to both dermatologists and primary care providers also requires creativity. As emphasized above, if workload increases for either or both services, incentives and support are critical for success. Benefits to primary care providers are often greatest in the New Service scenario. Providing education and quick consultative services to rural primary care physicians can be important motivators. Dermatologists and primary care providers must be involved in program planning from the outset to provide insight on the business model and workflow issues. It is also important to incorporate teledermatology into regular clinic procedures. For example, one teledermatology program failed, in part, simply because it took the dermatologist 15 minutes each way to walk to the telemedicine area.[86]

Provide Teledermatology Specific Training

The teledermatologist often provides hands on training for the teledermatology technician. Several helpful resources are available on dermatology-specific photography and recommended medical histories for teledermatology.[83,90,91,92] It is ideal if the teledermatology technician and local dermatology champion learn basic dermatology terminology, common skin conditions, and criteria for appropriate teledermatology consults. Periodic refresher training should also be included.

Table 11. Key Elements for Success and Barriers to Implementation

Facilitators for Implementation

Determine Relative Advantage
        Define objectives
        Evaluate alternatives to teledermatology
        Clarify if relative risk of implementation is manageable
        Conduct initial cost analysis and estimate

Assess Compatibility
        Involve all parties in the planning and implementation process
        Understand organization layout
        Obtain buy-in from key players
        Research resources available (primary care, specialty care, community)

Design Low Complexity System
        Create easy to use system
        Provide onsite technology support
        Provide support at referring site (technician/consult manager)
        Provide support for additional workload at dermatology site
        Incorporate teledermatology into usual processes
        Minimize patient waiting time

Ensure Trialability
        Reconceptualize professional roles/duties and ensure high levels of flexibility
        Provide training and feedback for teledermatology technician/consult manager
        Analyze business process and refine

Demonstrate Observability
        Determine if objectives are met, disseminate findings and evaluate improvement steps

Barriers to Implementation

Administrative:
        Lack of initial administrative support
        Lack of *ongoing* support

Clinical:
        Insufficient training of primary care and dermatology in use of teledermatology
        Single person trained who may not be available
        Inertia among potential users (patients, primary care, dermatology)
        Increased workload for primary care and dermatology without additional support
        Lack of clinical follow-up
        System does not fit objectives of the site
        Emphasis on technology rather than practical implementation and ongoing support

Patient:
        Patient inconvenience
        Lack of education of participants (patients and providers)
        Patient preference to see "in-person" dermatologist

Technical:
        Software problems
        Purchase of general teledermatology equipment rather than standard digital camera
        Poor photo quality
        Lack of standardization

SUMMARY AND DISCUSSION

This report summarizes a large body of evidence regarding: 1) teledermatology for the diagnosis of skin conditions, 2) teledermatology for the management of skin conditions, 3) clinical outcomes when teledermatology is used 4) the cost of teledermatology, and 5) key elements of and barriers to successful implementation of teledermatology. Differences in study settings, skin conditions, trial methodology, and outcomes weaken the strength of the evidence. When appropriate, we calculated weighted pooled estimates for similar studies. Summarized evidence indicates that diagnostic accuracy of usual care (in-person dermatology visit) is 5 to 19% (average absolute difference) better than teledermatology. When dermatoscopy-trained teledermatologists are available, teledermatoscopy improves diagnostic accuracy of circumscribed skin lesions, although generally not to a level exceeding usual care. We found that diagnostic and management concordance of usual care (in-person dermatology visit) and teledermatology is good for SAF and may be better for LI, likely due to the ability to obtain additional history in the LI setting. Limited data from two SAF studies, both from the same VA medical center, show that while overall management accuracy rates are equivalent for SF teledermatology and usual care, teledermatology is significantly less accurate for malignant skin lesions including squamous cell carcinoma, basal cell carcinoma, and melanoma. While this finding needs to be confirmed in other settings and in other study populations, awareness of this potential limitation of teledermatology in a VA population is important.

Our search found very little evidence on clinical course, an important limitation also noted in a 2006 report from the Agency for Healthcare Research and Quality (AHRQ).[95] Studies evaluating visits avoided uniformly showed that teledermatology can decrease the number of dermatology clinic visits. While studies of patient satisfaction were generally positive, factors such as distance to the dermatology clinic and wait times for an in-person appointment play important roles in patient satisfaction. Cost analyses were limited by broad variations in cost assessment parameters and perspectives. The majority of studies found teledermatology to be cost effective if certain critical assumptions were met; the most important included patient travel distance, teledermatology volume, and costs of usual care.

While evaluation of accuracy and reliability of a new technology is important, many more factors become important in evaluating clinical outcomes. Especially for SAF teledermatology, if recommendations are not communicated to the patient or not implemented by the referring provider, patient outcome is likely to be poor, despite a highly accurate and reliable technology. Because teledermatology involves a shift in workload, ongoing support (i.e., funding for a teledermatology technician, training for primary care physicians, additional dermatology staff) is critical. Barriers to implementation and key factors for success are highly dependent on the intended setting. Identifying site-specific barriers is critical to successful implementation.

CONCLUSIONS

In general, diagnostic accuracy of usual care (in-person dermatology care) is better than SAF teledermatology. Both SAF as well as LI teledermatology appear to have acceptable diagnostic and concordance compared to clinic dermatology. SAF is currently more widely used in the VA. Little information exists on the impact of teledermatology on clinical outcomes and management compared to management provided by in clinic dermatologists. This may be particularly important for dermatologic conditions with potentially serious outcomes (e.g., malignant and premalignant lesions). Patient satisfaction with teledermatology is relatively high though there are individuals who have strong beliefs for a particular approach and little information exists from non-research settings regarding patient satisfaction. Cost analysis studies are limited in number and relevance to current VA practice. Identifying and removing barriers to successful implementation is essential. Studies are needed to compare teledermatology with primary care to inform decision making about the best way to provide dermatology in areas without reliable access to in-person dermatology (e.g., rural areas). Given the results of this review, the potential benefits of teledermatology (e.g., decreased patient travel, shorter time to intervention, primary care provider education) need to be evaluated in the context of its limitations including inferior diagnostic accuracy and management accuracy, especially for malignant skin neoplasms.

FUTURE RESEARCH RECOMMENDATIONS

Additional research is needed to determine the long-term effectiveness, feasibility, satisfaction, and cost-effectiveness of teledermatology (especially store and forward methodologies) integrated into primary care settings with outcomes related to the impact of teledermatology on patient management and clinical outcomes. Standardized reporting of diagnostic, management, and outcome accuracy and concordance are needed. Future studies should attempt to distinguish between lack of concordance between two in-person dermatologists and lack of concordance between teledermatology and in-person dermatology. Studies that blind assessors to the patient/lesion are preferred to reduce bias in outcome assessment. Additional outcomes could assess the impact on primary care practice, referring provider satisfaction, and follow-up patterns. Barriers to successful implementation need to be identified that incorporate differences in patient populations, lesion severity, and acuteness; distance traveled and availability of local dermatologists; and other clinical setting issues in order to determine the relative feasibility and effectiveness of different teledermatology strategies in different settings (e.g., Intrasite, Intersite, New Site).

Importantly, while this review suggests that diagnostic accuracy of teledermatology is inferior to in-person dermatologic care, teledermatology may still be superior to dermatologic care provided by a non-dermatologist; studies are needed to compare teledermatology with primary care. Additional research is needed to determine the long-term outcomes and cost-effectiveness of teledermatology (especially store and forward methodology) in the VA setting. We are aware of one randomized controlled study in progress (Impact of Teledermatology on Health Services Outcomes in the VA HSRD IIR05-278, PI John Whited) which will assess quality of life and nine-month clinical course outcomes in two VA SAF teledermatology programs.

We recommend prioritizing studies which address the following outcomes:

1. Comparison of teledermatology with dermatologic care by a VA primary care provider or a dermatology trained nurse practitioner: This study setting is very relevant to remote/inaccessible locations where no in-person dermatologist is available (e.g., Hawaii, Alaska, remote rural clinics). Relevant outcomes include diagnostic accuracy and concordance, management accuracy and concordance, long-term outcomes, cost-effectiveness, and patient/provider satisfaction.

2. Comparison of teledermatology with in-person care by a dermatologist in a VA setting: Long-term clinical outcomes, patient and provider satisfaction, and cost analyses are needed. Additional outcomes should assess the impact of teledermatology on primary care practice and follow-up patterns. Barriers to successful implementation need to be identified that incorporate differences in patient populations, skin condition severity and acuteness, distance traveled, and availability of on-site dermatologists.

3. Comparison of specific imaging techniques to enhance teledermatology accuracy: More research is needed to understand the limitations of teledermatology (e.g., malignant skin neoplasms) and whether specific techniques (e.g., polarized light dermatoscopy, contact immersion dermatoscopy, and confocal microscopy) can overcome these limitations.

4. Evaluation of teledermatology to provide follow-up dermatologic care: Clinical outcomes, feasibility, and cost analyses are needed to evaluate chronic skin conditions which require frequent monitoring such as leg ulcers, post-operative wound care, and chronic dermatitis.

REFERENCES

1.   Oakley A, Rademaker M, Duffill M. Teledermatology in the Waikato region of New Zealand. Journal of Telemedicine & Telecare 2001; 7 Suppl 2:59-61.

2.   Rogers EM. Diffusion of innovations. New York: The Free Press, 1995.

3.   Greenhalgh T, Robert G, Bate P, Macfarlane F, Kyriakidou O. Diffusion of innovations in health service organizations: a systematic literature review. Malden, MA: Blackwell Publishing Ltd., 2005.

4.   Whiting P, Rutjes AWS, Reitsma JB, Bossuyt PMM, Kleijnen J. The development of QUADAS: a tool for the quality assessment of studies of diagnostic accuracy included in systematic reviews. BMC Medical Research Methodology 2003;3:25 (available at http://www.biomedcentral.com/1471-2288/3/25.

5.   Warshaw EM, Lederle FA, Grill JP, et al. Accuracy of teledermatology for pigmented neoplasms. Journal of the American Academy of Dermatology 2009; 61:753-765.

6.   Warshaw EM, Lederle FA, Grill JP, et al. Accuracy of teledermatology for nonpigmented neoplasms. Journal of the American Academy of Dermatology 2009; 60(4):579-88.

7.   Edison KE, Ward DS, Dyer JA, et al. Diagnosis, diagnostic confidence, and management concordance in live interactive and store-and-forward teledermatology compared to in-person examination. Telemedicine Journal & E-Health 2008; 14(9):889-95.

8.   Fabbrocini G, Balato A, Rescigno O, et al. Telediagnosis and face-to-face diagnosis reliability for melanocytic and non-melanocytic 'pink' lesions. Journal of the European Academy of Dermatology & Venereology 2008; 22(2):229-34.

9.   Di Stefani A, Zalaudek I, Argenziano G, et al. Feasibility of a two-step teledermatologic approach for the management of patients with multiple pigmented skin lesions. Dermatologic Surgery 2007; 33(6):686-92.

10.   Ferrandiz L, Moreno-Ramirez D, Nieto-Garcia A, et al. Teledermatology-based presurgical management for nonmelanoma skin cancer: a pilot study. Dermatologic Surgery 2007; 33(9):1092-8.

11.   Moreno-Ramirez D, Ferrandiz L, Nieto-Garcia A, et al. Store-and-forward teledermatology in skin cancer triage: experience and evaluation of 2009 teleconsultations. Archives of Dermatology 2007; 143(4):479-84.

12.   Bowns IR, Collins K, Walters SJ, et al. Telemedicine in dermatology: a randomised controlled trial. Health Technology Assessment 2006; 10(43):3-25.

13.   Bowns IR, Collins K, Walters SJ, et al. Telemedicine in dermatology: a randomised controlled trial. Health Technology Assessment 2006; 10(43):27-33.

14.   Moreno-Ramirez D, Ferrandiz L, Galdeano R, et al. Teledermatoscopy as a triage system for pigmented lesions: a pilot study. Clinical & Experimental Dermatology 2006; 31(1):13-8.

15. Oakley AM, Reeves F, Bennett J, et al. Diagnostic value of written referral and/or images for skin lesions. Journal of Telemedicine & Telecare 2006; 12(3):151-8.

16. Mahendran R, Goodfield MJ, Sheehan-Dare RA. An evaluation of the role of a store-and-forward teledermatology system in skin cancer diagnosis and management. Clinical & Experimental Dermatology 2005; 30(3):209-14.

17. Baba M, Seckin D, Kapdagli S. A comparison of teledermatology using store-and-forward methodology alone, and in combination with Web camera videoconferencing. Journal of Telemedicine & Telecare 2005; 11(7):354-60.

18. Moreno-Ramirez D, Ferrandiz L, Bernal AP, et al. Teledermatology as a filtering system in pigmented lesion clinics. Journal of Telemedicine & Telecare 2005; 11(6):298-303.

19. Tucker WF, Lewis FM. Digital imaging: a diagnostic screening tool? International Journal of Dermatology 2005; 44(6):479-81.

20. Oztas MO, Calikoglu E, Baz K, et al. Reliability of Web-based teledermatology consultations. Journal of Telemedicine & Telecare 2004; 10(1):25-8.

21. Ferrara G, Argenziano G, Cerroni L, et al. A pilot study of a combined dermoscopic-pathological approach to the telediagnosis of melanocytic skin neoplasms. Journal of Telemedicine & Telecare 2004; 10(1):34-8.

22. Piccolo D, Soyer HP, Chimenti S, et al. Diagnosis and categorization of acral melanocytic lesions using teledermoscopy. Journal of Telemedicine & Telecare 2004; 10(6):346-50.

23. Shapiro M, James WD, Kessler R, et al. Comparison of skin biopsy triage decisions in 49 patients with pigmented lesions and skin neoplasms: store-and-forward teledermatology vs face-to-face dermatology. Archives of Dermatology 2004; 140(5):525-8.

24. Coras B, Glaessl A, Kinateder J, et al. Teledermatoscopy in daily routine--results of the first 100 cases. Current Problems in Dermatology 2003; 32:207-12.

25. Du Moulin MF, Bullens-Goessens YI, Henquet CJ, et al. The reliability of diagnosis using store-and-forward teledermatology. Journal of Telemedicine & Telecare 2003; 9(5):249-52.

26. Pak HS, Harden D, Cruess D, et al. Teledermatology: an intraobserver diagnostic correlation study, Part II. Cutis 2003; 71(6):476-80.

27. Pak HS, Harden D, Cruess D, et al. Teledermatology: an intraobserver diagnostic correlation study, Part I. Cutis 2003; 71(5):399-403.

28. Rashid E, Ishtiaq O, Gilani S, et al. Comparison of store and forward method of teledermatology with face-to-face consultation. Journal of Ayub Medical College, Abbottabad: JAMC 2003; 15(2):34-6.

29.   Oliveira MR, Wen CL, Neto CF, et al. Web site for training nonmedical health-care work-
      ers to identify potentially malignant skin lesions and for teledermatology. Telemedicine
      Journal & E-Health 2002; 8(3):323-32.

30.   Jolliffe VM, Harris DW, Whittaker SJ. Can we safely diagnose pigmented lesions from
      stored video images? A diagnostic comparison between clinical examination and stored
      video images of pigmented lesions removed for histology. Clinical & Experimental Der-
      matology 2001; 26(1):84-7.

31.   Jolliffe VM, Harris DW, Morris R, et al. Can we use video images to triage pigmented
      lesions? British Journal of Dermatology 2001; 145(6):904-10.

32.   Lim AC, Egerton IB, See A, et al. Accuracy and reliability of store-and-forward teleder-
      matology: preliminary results from the St George Teledermatology Project. Australasian
      Journal of Dermatology 2001; 42(4):247-51.

33.   Taylor P, Goldsmith P, Murray K, et al. Evaluating a telemedicine system to assist in the
      management of dermatology referrals. British Journal of Dermatology 2001; 144(2):328-
      33.

34.   Barnard CM, Goldyne ME. Evaluation of an asynchronous teleconsultation system for
      diagnosis of skin cancer and other skin diseases. Telemedicine Journal & E-Health 2000;
      6(4):379-84.

35.   Braun RP, Meier M, Pelloni F, et al. Teledermatoscopy in Switzerland: a preliminary
      evaluation. Journal of the American Academy of Dermatology 2000; 42(5 Pt 1):770-5.

36.   High WA, Houston MS, Calobrisi SD, et al. Assessment of the accuracy of low-cost
      store-and-forward teledermatology consultation. Journal of the American Academy of
      Dermatology 2000; 42(5 Pt 1):776-83.

37.   Piccolo D, Smolle J, Argenziano G, et al. Teledermoscopy--results of a multicentre study
      on 43 pigmented skin lesions. Journal of Telemedicine & Telecare 2000; 6(3):132-7.

38.   Krupinski EA, LeSueur B, Ellsworth L, et al. Diagnostic accuracy and image quality us-
      ing a digital camera for teledermatology. Telemedicine Journal 1999; 5(3):257-63.

39.   Lewis K, Gilmour E, Harrison PV, et al. Digital teledermatology for skin tumours: a pre-
      liminary assessment using a receiver operating characteristics (ROC) analysis. Journal of
      Telemedicine & Telecare 1999; 5 Suppl 1:S57-8.

40.   Piccolo D, Smolle J, Wolf IH, et al. Face-to-face diagnosis vs telediagnosis of pigmented
      skin tumors: a teledermoscopic study. Archives of Dermatology 1999; 135(12):1467-71.

41.   Tait CP, Clay CD. Pilot study of store and forward teledermatology services in Perth,
      Western Australia. Australasian Journal of Dermatology 1999; 40(4):190-3.

42.   Whited JD, Hall RP, Simel DL, et al. Reliability and accuracy of dermatologists' clinic-
      based and digital image consultations. Journal of the American Academy of Dermatology
      1999; 41(5 Pt 1):693-702.

43. Whited JD, Mills BJ, Hall RP, et al. A pilot trial of digital imaging in skin cancer. Journal of Telemedicine & Telecare 1998; 4(2):108-12.

44. Kvedar JC, Edwards RA, Menn ER, et al. The substitution of digital images for dermatologic physical examination. Archives of Dermatology 1997; 133(2):161-7.

45. Lyon CC, Harrison PV. A portable digital imaging system in dermatology: diagnostic and educational applications. Journal of Telemedicine & Telecare 1997; 3 Suppl 1:81-3.

46. Zelickson BD, Homan L. Teledermatology in the nursing home. Archives of Dermatology 1997; 133(2):171-4.

47. Nordal EJ, Moseng D, Kvammen B, et al. A comparative study of teleconsultations versus face-to-face consultations. Journal of Telemedicine & Telecare 2001; 7(5):257-65.

48. Gilmour E, Campbell SM, Loane MA, et al. Comparison of teleconsultations and face-to-face consultations: preliminary results of a United Kingdom multicentre teledermatology study. British Journal of Dermatology 1998; 139(1):81-7.

49. Lesher JL, Jr., Davis LS, Gourdin FW, et al. Telemedicine evaluation of cutaneous diseases: a blinded comparative study. Journal of the American Academy of Dermatology 1998; 38(1):27-31.

50. Loane MA, Corbett R, Bloomer SE, et al. Diagnostic accuracy and clinical management by realtime teledermatology. Results from the Northern Ireland arms of the UK Multicentre Teledermatology Trial. Journal of Telemedicine & Telecare 1998; 4(2):95-100.

51. Lowitt MH, Kessler, II, Kauffman CL, et al. Teledermatology and in-person examinations: a comparison of patient and physician perceptions and diagnostic agreement. Archives of Dermatology 1998; 134(4):471-6.

52. Phillips CM, Burke WA, Allen MH, et al. Reliability of telemedicine in evaluating skin tumors. Telemedicine Journal 1998; 4(1):5-9.

53. Oakley AM, Astwood DR, Loane M, et al. Diagnostic accuracy of teledermatology: results of a preliminary study in New Zealand. New Zealand Medical Journal 1997; 110(1038):51-3.

54. Phillips CM, Burke WA, Shechter A, et al. Reliability of dermatology teleconsultations with the use of teleconferencing technology. Journal of the American Academy of Dermatology 1997; 37(3 Pt 1):398-402.

55. Warshaw EM, Gravely AA, Nelson DB. Accuracy of Teledermatology/Teledermatoscopy and Clinical-Based Dermatology for Specific Categories of Skin Neoplasms. Submitted to Journal of the American Academy of Dermatology (JAAD) on 9-9-09 JAAD-D-09-0124, resubmitted 10-9-09, accepted 10-30-09.

56. Loane MA, Gore HE, Bloomer SE, et al. Preliminary results from the Northern Ireland arms of the UK Multicentre Teledermatology Trial: is clinical management by realtime teledermatology possible? Journal of Telemedicine & Telecare 1998; 4 Suppl 1:3-5.

57.   Eminovic N, de Keizer NF, Wyatt JC, et al. Teledermatologic consultation and reduction in referrals to dermatologists: a cluster randomized controlled trial. Archives of Dermatology 2009; 145(5):558-64.

58.   Pak H, Triplett CA, Lindquist JH, et al. Store-and-forward teledermatology results in similar clinical outcomes to conventional clinic-based care. Journal of Telemedicine & Telecare 2007; 13(1):26-30.

59.   Granlund H, Thoden CJ, Carlson C, et al. Realtime teleconsultations versus face-to-face consultations in dermatology: immediate and six-month outcome. Journal of Telemedicine & Telecare 2003; 9(4):204-9.

60.   Whited JD, Hall RP, Foy ME, et al. Patient and clinician satisfaction with a store-and-forward teledermatology consult system. Telemedicine Journal & E-Health 2004; 10(4):422-31.

61.   Weinstock MA, Nguyen FQ, Risica PM. Patient and referring provider satisfaction with teledermatology. Journal of the American Academy of Dermatology 2002; 47(1):68-72.

62.   Williams TL, Esmail A, May CR, et al. Patient satisfaction with teledermatology is related to perceived quality of life. British Journal of Dermatology 2001; 145(6):911-7.

63.   Williams TL, Esmail A, May CR, et al. Patient satisfaction with store-and-forward teledermatology. Journal of Telemedicine & Telecare 2001; 7 Suppl 1:45-6.

64.   Pak HS, Welch M, Poropatich R. Web-based teledermatology consult system: preliminary results from the first 100 cases. Studies in Health Technology & Informatics 1999; 64:179-84.

65.   Hicks LL, Boles KE, Hudson S, et al. Patient satisfaction with teledermatology services. Journal of Telemedicine & Telecare 2003; 9(1):42-5.

66.   Lamminen H, Tuomi ML, Lamminen J, et al. A feasibility study of realtime teledermatology in Finland. Journal of Telemedicine & Telecare 2000; 6(2):102-7.

67.   Loane MA, Bloomer SE, Corbett R, et al. Patient satisfaction with realtime teledermatology in Northern Ireland. Journal of Telemedicine & Telecare 1998; 4(1):36-40.

68.   Hsiao JL, Oh DH. The impact of store-and-forward teledermatology on skin cancer diagnosis and treatment. Journal of the American Academy of Dermatology 2008; 59(2):260-7.

69.   Whited JD, Hall RP, Foy ME, et al. Teledermatology's impact on time to intervention among referrals to a dermatology consult service. Telemedicine Journal & E-Health 2002; 8(3):313-21.

70.   Loane MA, Bloomer SE, Corbett R, et al. A randomized controlled trial assessing the health economics of realtime teledermatology compared with conventional care: an urban versus rural perspective. Journal of Telemedicine & Telecare 2001; 7(2):108-18.

71.   Wootton R, Bloomer SE, Corbett R, et al. Multicentre randomised control trial comparing real time teledermatology with conventional outpatient dermatological care: societal cost-benefit analysis. BMJ 2000; 320(7244):1252-6.

72.   Knol A, van den Akker TW, Damstra RJ, et al. Teledermatology reduces the number of patient referrals to a dermatologist. Journal of Telemedicine & Telecare 2006; 12(2):75-8.

73.   Whited JD, Datta S, Hall RP, et al. An economic analysis of a store and forward teledermatology consult system. Telemedicine Journal & E-Health 2003; 9(4):351-60.

74.   Pak HS, Datta SK, Triplett CA, et al. Cost minimization analysis of a store-and-forward teledermatology consult system. Telemedicine Journal & E-Health 2009; 15(2):160-5.

75.   Moreno-Ramirez D, Ferrandiz L, Ruiz-de-Casas A, et al. Economic evaluation of a store-and-forward teledermatology system for skin cancer patients. Journal of Telemedicine & Telecare 2009; 15(1):40-5.

76.   Burgiss SG, Julius CE, Watson HW, et al. Telemedicine for dermatology care in rural patients. Telemedicine Journal 1997; 3(3):227-33.

77.   Loane MA, Oakley A, Rademaker M, et al. A cost-minimization analysis of the societal costs of realtime teledermatology compared with conventional care: results from a randomized controlled trial in New Zealand. Journal of Telemedicine & Telecare 2001; 7(4):233-8.

78.   Bergmo TS. A cost-minimization analysis of a realtime teledermatology service in northern Norway. Journal of Telemedicine & Telecare 2000; 6(5):273-7.

79.   Armstrong AW, Dorer DJ, Lugn NE, et al. Economic evaluation of interactive teledermatology compared with conventional care. Telemedicine Journal & E-Health 2007; 13(2):91-9.

80.   Loane MA, Bloomer SE, Corbett R, et al. A comparison of real-time and store-and-forward teledermatology: a cost-benefit study. British Journal of Dermatology 2000; 143(6):1241-7.

81.   English JS, Eedy DJ. Has teledermatology in the U.K. finally failed? British Journal of Dermatology 2007; 156(3):411.

82.   Finch TL, Mair FS, May CR. Teledermatology in the UK: lessons in service innovation. British Journal of Dermatology 2007; 156(3):521-7.

83.   Pak HS. Implementing a teledermatology programme. Journal of Telemedicine & Telecare 2005; 11(6):285-93.

84.   Stronge AJ, Nichols T, Rogers WA, et al. Systematic human factors evaluation of a teledermatology system within the U.S. military. Telemedicine Journal & E-Health 2008; 14(1):25-34.

85.   Pak HS. Teledermatology and teledermatopathology. Seminars in Cutaneous Medicine & Surgery 2002; 21(3):179-89.

86.   Carlos ME, Pangelinan SI. Teledermatology in Department of Defense Health Services Region 10. Journal of Healthcare Information Management 1999; 13(4):59-69.

87.   Finch T. Teledermatology for chronic disease management: coherence and normalization. Chronic Illness 2008; 4(2):127-34.

88.   Pak H. Teledermatology in North America. Current Problems in Dermatology 2003; 32:222-5.

89.   See A, Lim AC, Le K, et al. Operational teledermatology in Broken Hill, rural Australia. Australasian Journal of Dermatology 2005; 46(3):144-9.

90.   Krupinski E, Burdick A, Pak Hon, et al. Practice Guidelines for Teledermatology, December 2007. Available at: http://www.americantelemed.org/files/public/standards/Telederm_guidelines_v10final_withCOVER.pdf. Accessed November, 2009.

91.   Vidmar DA. The Idiot's Guide to Teledermatology Imaging. Available at: www.healthcare.hqusareur.army.mil/Telemedicine2004.02.04/Pubs/Telederm.pdf. Accessed November, 2009.

92.   VHA Telehealth Operations Manual for Teledermatology, Revision July 30, 2008;. Available at: http://vaww.carecoordination.va.gov/store-forward/teledermatology/. Accesssed November, 2009.

93.   van den Akker TW, Reker CH, Knol A, et al. Teledermatology as a tool for communication between general practitioners and dermatologists. Journal of Telemedicine & Telecare 2001; 7(4):193-8.

94.   Collins K, Bowns I, Walters S. General practitioners' perceptions of asynchronous telemedicine in a randomized controlled trial of teledermatology. Journal of Telemedicine & Telecare 2004;10(2):94-98.

95.   Hersh WR, Hickam DH, Severance SM, Dana TL, Krages KP, Helfand M. Telemedicine for the Medicare Population: Update. Evidence Report/Technology Assessment No. 131 (Prepared by the Oregon Evidence-based Practice Center under Contract No. 290-02-0024.) AHRQ Publication No. 06-E007. Rockville, MD: Agency for Healthcare Research and Quality. February, 2006.

APPENDIX A. SEARCH STRATEGY

Database: Ovid MEDLINE(R) <1950 to April Week 3 2009>

Search Strategy:

----

1   (remote: adj2 consult:).tw. (158)

2   exp electronic mail/ (1025)

3   exp Telecommunications/ (36778)

4   exp remote consultation/ (2661)

5   telemed$.mp. or exp Telemedicine/ (10571)

6   exp telepathology/ (504)

7   or/1-6 (37311)

8   derm$.mp. or exp dermatology/ (180688)

9   7 and 8 (534)

10   telederm$.mp. (269)

11   9 or 10 (576)

12   limit 11 to yr="1990 -Current" (559)

PubMed search (06-03-09):

(((remote* AND consult*[tw]) OR (electronic mail[mh]) OR (telecommunications[mh]) OR (remote consultation[mh]) OR (telemed* OR telemedicine[mh]) OR (telepathology[mh])) AND (dermatol* OR dermatology[mh])) OR (telederm*) [587]

Search results from OVID MEDLINE (556 references) and PubMed (587 references) were combined, resulting in a total of 657 unique references

APPENDIX B. DATA EXTRACTION FORM

First author: _____

Year published: _____

Country where study performed (country of first author or multicenter): _____

Source of funding for study: _____

Extractor: _____

DESIGN (circle):

Systematic review   Cross-sectional study

Randomized controlled clinical trial   Case series

Non-randomized controlled clinical trial   Case report

Cohort study   Qualitative

Case-control study   Editorial/opinion piece/letter

Other evaluation of diagnostic test

KEY QUESTION(S) (circle):

KQ1: Diagnostic accuracy/reliability

KQ2: Clinical management accuracy/reliability

KQ3: Clinical outcomes (clinical course, satisfaction, quality of life, visits avoided, etc.)

KQ4: Costs

KQ5: Implementation

Background

NOTES:

□ Study contains/may contain same data as another study (specify study: _____

_____)

STUDY SETTING/EQUIPMENT:

Single- or Multi-center trial?   (*circle one*)

      a. # of sites where photos obtained _____

      setting for each site (e.g., patient home, physician office, hospital, nursing home, etc.)

          1.

          2.

          3.

          4.

      b. # of sites where photos interpreted _____

      setting for each site (e.g., dermatology clinic [or other type of clinic], hospital, VA or non-VA, academic or community-based, etc.)

          1.

          2.

          3.

          4.

Technology used: Store & Forward   Live Interactive

Purpose of examination: Diagnosis   Therapy   Follow-up   Other _____

Camera type: _____   Pixels: _____

Special imaging technique(s) (describe): _____

_____

Image interpretation technique(s): _____

_____

PROVIDERS (e.g., family practice dermatologist, specialist dermatologist, dermatopathologist):

A. Gold Standard Test Provider

1.   Clinical dermatologist (in-person evaluation)
        Level of training
        Experience with teledermatology (volume of cases, if reported)

2.   Histodermatologist
        Level of training
        Experience with teledermatology (volume of cases, if reported)

B. Index Test Provider
        Level of training
        Experience with teledermatology (volume of cases, if reported)

C. Photographer/History Taker (if different from Index Test Provider)
        Level of training
        Experience with teledermatology (volume of cases, if reported)

STUDY PARTICIPANTS:

Number enrolled: _____

How were patients recruited? _____

Inclusion Criteria: _____

Exclusion Criteria: _____

Age   Mean _____ yrs   Range _____ yrs

Gender   Female _____ %   Male _____ %

Veterans   _____ %

Race (describe) _____

Other population characteristics (describe): _____

_____

Number of lesions/conditions evaluated: _____

Dermatologic condition(s): Rash _____   Lesion _____   Mixed _____

        Other details about condition(s), if provided _____

Gold standard: In-person Dermatology _____   Histopathology _____
                  Other (specify) _____

STUDY FEATURES/QUALITY:

FOR DIAGNOSTIC ACCURACY TESTS (Yes, No, Unclear):

(NOTE: index test is new, unproven test; gold standard is established reference test)

	Y	N	U
1. Study patients representative of actual patient population to be tested	Y	N	U
2. Inclusion/exclusion criteria clearly described	Y	N	U
3. Appropriate (accurate) gold standard	Y	N	U
4. Time between index and gold standard assessments appropriate (i.e., insufficient time for disease progression or recovery)	Y	N	U
5. All (or random sample) of patients received both tests	Y	N	U
6. Same gold standard used for all patients	Y	N	U
7. Gold standard independent of index test	Y	N	U
8. Sufficient detail provided to replicate index test	Y	N	U
9. Sufficient detail provided to replicate gold standard test	Y	N	U
10. Index test interpreted without knowledge of gold standard results	Y	N	U
11. Gold standard interpreted without knowledge of index results	Y	N	U
12. Similar clinical data available during test interpretation as in practice	Y	N	U
13. Uninterpretable/indeterminate test results reported (i.e., all test results reported)	Y	N	U
14. All patients accounted for at end of study	Y	N	U

FOR CONTROLLED TRIALS (Yes, No, Unclear, Not Applicable) (adapted from USPSTF approach):

1. Initial assembly of comparable groups
   a. Randomized trials

True randomization	Y	N	U	NA
Concealment	Y	N	U	NA

b. Other studies

Inclusion/exclusion criteria defined and applied to all groups	Y	N	U	NA
Potential confounders considered	Y	N	U	NA

2. Groups similar at baseline   Y   N   U   NA

      If not, describe significant differences _____

3. Comparable groups maintained (attrition, cross-overs,   Y   N   U   NA
         adherence, etc.)

     Loss to follow-up (%): _____

     If not comparable for all groups, explain: _____

4. Blinding (masking)

a. Participants	Y	N	U	NA
b. Outcome Assessment	Y	N	U	NA

5. All important outcomes considered   Y   N   U   NA

6. Outcome measures reliable and valid   Y   N   U   NA

7. Analysis

a.   RCT – Intention-to-treat   Y   N   U   NA

    b.   Other – confounders adjusted for, if needed   Y   N   U   NA

RESULTS:

Number of patients with complete data: _____

Reasons for incomplete data: _____

Significant differences between patients enrolled and patients who completed study? _____
_____

Time between photograph and gold-standard interpretation of condition (mean and/or range): _____

Length of follow-up (for follow-up studies only): _____

Study duration: _____

FOR STUDIES THAT REPORT SENSITIVITY AND SPECIFICITY:

Complete the following table if possible (see definitions at end of form):

		Reference (Gold Standard) Test Findings		
		Positive	Negative	
Index Test Findings	Positive			PPV=
	Negative			NPV=
		Sens.=	Spec.=	

OTHER AGREEMENT OUTCOMES:

Kappa Coefficient: _____

Percent Agreement: _____

Other Outcomes (describe): _____

_____

CLINICAL MANAGEMENT OUTCOMES:

Clinical course (describe outcomes):

Patient satisfaction with teledermatology (assessment tool, outcomes):

Quality of life (assessment tool, outcomes):

Clinic visits avoided? Yes (# if provided _____) No

Did test results influence treatment selected for patients?
Describe: _____

_____

_____

Did test results influence management strategy for patients?

Describe: _____

_____

_____

OTHER RELEVANT FINDINGS:

AUTHORS' CONCLUSIONS:

APPENDIX C. PEER REVIEW COMMENTS AND AUTHOR RESPONSES

REVIEWER COMMENT	RESPONSE
1. Are the objectives, scope, and methods for this review clearly described?	
Yes	NA
Yes	NA
2. Is there any indication of bias in our synthesis of the evidence?	
No	NA
No	NA
3. Are there any published or <u>unpublished</u> studies on the use of teledermatology for the diagnosis and management of skin conditions (including studies of clinical outcomes, patient satisfaction, or associated costs) that we may have overlooked?	
None that I am aware of	NA
None that I'm aware of	NA
4. Additional comments	
The current format serves as a comprehensive review of the status of the literature.	Thank you
Quality of teledermatology – how is the quality of the test itself ensured?	We assume the reviewer is asking about the quality of the picture image. We did not specifically look at image techniques but we only included studies published after 1990 to insure technical relevance.
EXECUTIVE SUMMARY:	
In the summary for KQ4, clarify the statement "The long duration to achieve definitive dermatologic care … is not consistent with current VA practice …"	We have clarified this statement.
In the executive summary I would prefer to see the Key Question stated followed by the conclusion. Following that, there could be the brief discussion of the results from the literature (that supports that conclusion).	Thank you for the suggestion. We have placed the conclusions immediately following the questions.
In "Methods" state that all-pediatric studies were excluded	To shorten the Executive Summary, we have deleted the inclusion/exclusion details. We have clarified the inclusion/exclusion criteria for studies in the full report.
KQ3 – Clarify the "clinical outcomes of interest"	We have specified the outcomes of interest.

Comment	Response
Conclusion – As worded, the conclusion may be misinterpreted as overly negative; the true comparison needed for many populations is between telederm and primary care diagnosis and management	We agree that this type of study is needed and have clarified the conclusion statements to reflect that.
Interpretation of 'raw' comparisons – I'm not sure what it means that 'weighted mean absolute difference was 19% better for UC than teledermatology' (page v) – perhaps include some concrete examples to make the numbers more meaningful or at least place them in some context (e.g., for other comparisons of diagnostic tests)	These comparisons have been reworded to clarify that these differences are differences in accuracy rates.
Define abbreviations before using them	We have made this change.
Not sure why inclusion was limited to randomized trials for questions 1-2; does this mean that retrospective reviews of telederm consults were not included? (page iii)	Inclusion was for controlled trials (not randomized); most were repeated measure design. Retrospective reviews were included if a control group was utilized. This has been clarified in the inclusion/exclusion criteria.
Did teledermoscopy improve accuracy of teledermatology to *better* than UC, or at least much closer? (page v)	This statement has been revised to clarify that accuracy improved, but still was not better than usual care.
Conclusion should probably include the information that the accuracy and concordance for malignancies may not be acceptable (page xlvii)	This information has been added.
INTRODUCTION/BACKGROUND:	
Do you have data to support the statement "SAF is the more widely used form of teledermatology in the VA"?	An informal survey of dermatology chiefs is included in the introduction.
METHODS:	
On the literature flow diagram, clarify the "other" and "not eligible study setting" exclusion criteria	We have modified the study exclusion criteria, eliminating these two criteria.
List the inclusion and exclusion criteria for studies (bulleted format)	These have been reformatted into bullet structure.
Inclusion/exclusion criteria – could have used more explanation	These are now described.
Clarify the asterisk on the search results (657 references)	The explanation was inadvertently deleted from the draft sent for review; please see updated flow diagram.
Clarify why 1990 was chosen as the start date for the review	This has been clarified in the text.
Difficult for the reader to interpret the QUADAS scores – how do these compare with, say, the quality scores of primary studies in other systematic reviews?	There is no direct comparison. The QUADAS scale is, however, the most relevant for assessing the quality of studies of diagnostic tests.
RESULTS:	
Did we compare US vs. non-US studies? Do the results vary?	The results of the US vs. non-US studies were similar. We have revised the results section putting more emphasis on VA/DoD studies.
KQ2a – the conclusion is based on two studies from one center; it may be worth noting that the result may be hard to generalize to other health care setting/populations in active programs	This information has been added.
KQ5 – "Several publications have described …" – please make sure you include the VA Teledermatology Ops Manual	The references for this statement have been clarified – the Ops Manual is cited.

Comment	Response
KQ5 – "Because store and forward is the method used … " – I don't think this is true based on coding data	An e-mail survey of chiefs of VA dermatology services was conducted to confirm that SAF is more commonly used than LI in the VA setting.
CONCLUSIONS:	
Make the conclusions relevant to VA dermatology – readily usable by policy makers and clinicians	The conclusion section has been revised to focus on VA relevance.
How do the findings apply to situations with no available in-person dermatology? Is it possible to group studies based on the setting (very rural and urban)?	The conclusion section has been revised to address this.
FUTURE RESEARCH:	
Emphasize gaps in the current research – be specific, prioritize	The future research section has been been revised to address specific needed study outcomes and settings.
OVERALL:	
Consider changing the title to indicate that report is focused on adult population	Twenty of the included studies enrolled a mixed (adult/pediatric) population; it would not be possible to report only the results from the adults included in those trials.
A particular strength of this review is the overall framework that examines the diagnostic test(s) 'teledermatology' with respect to measurement characteristics, effects on patient care processes and outcomes, and organizational features related to successful implementation	Thank you.
The quality of this review is high in that it is clear, accurate, completed, and clinically relevant … the study questions were well-defined and important, the literature search appeared comprehensive, the methods of abstraction were adequate, judgments of methodological quality were included, the pooling of results seemed sensible and conservative, and the conclusions were reasonable.	Thank you.
No reference is made to the 2006 AHRQ Telemedicine review that covered teledermatology.	This reference has been added to the Summary and Discussion section.
It is usually acknowledged that there is a lack of concordance between face-to-face dermatology consultations and the difference between face-to-face and teledermatology is usually couched in this context.	A statement has been added to the Future Research Recommendations section.
Programs usually acknowledge the issues with pigmented lesions and expedite referral for these with teledermatology (a "triage" in which pigmented lesions and suspected malignancies are seen more rapidly)	We have noted the inferior management accuracy rates for malignant and pre-malignant lesions in our conclusion statements for Key Question 2 and in the Conclusions Section.
It is not clear whether the differences noted in the studies result in altered clinical outcomes for patients or are hypothetical.	We agree. As noted in the results for Key Question 3, there are few studies that directly address clinical outcomes.
Given the profound challenges with providing dermatology, especially in rural areas, issue of access are often that of teledermatology versus a general practitioner – this was alluded to but more emphasis could be placed on the issues with providing face-to-face dermatology nationwide.	We have added the need for research of this nature to the Conclusion section.
A further model of teledermatology is that of using a dermatology trained nurse practitioner.	None of the studies identified for the review evaluated this model. The need to include dermatology trained nurse practitioners was added to the Future Research section.

APPENDIX D. ABBREVIATIONS

CD =   Clinic dermatology/clinic dermatologist; in-person dermatology care/in-person dermatologist

CID =   Contact immersion dermatoscopy

DoD =   Department of Defense

DSC =   Dermatoscopy

Hrs =   Hours

k =   Kappa coefficient

KC=   Keratinocyte Carcinoma (BCC, SCC, Keratoacanthoma, SCC-in-situ)

KQ=   Key question

LI =   Live interactive teledermatology

95%CI =   95 percent confidence intervals

NPSL=   Non-pigmented skin lesions

NA=   Not applicable

NR =   Not reported

PLD =   Polarized light dermatoscopy

PSL =   Pigmented skin lesions

Pt =   Patient

RCT =   Randomized controlled trial

QUADAS =   Quality Assessment of Diagnostic Accuracy Studies

SAF =   Store and forward teledermatology

SD =   Standard deviation

SL =   Skin lesions

TD =   Teledermatology/teledermatologist

TDSC =   Teledermatoscopy

UC =   Usual care (in-person dermatology)

VA =   Veterans Affairs

vs. =   Versus

APPENDIX E. EVIDENCE TABLE
OVERVIEW OF STUDIES FOR KEY QUESTIONS 1 AND 2

Diagnostic Accuracy, Diagnostic Concordance, Management Accuracy, Management Concordance

Study Country Study design Funding	# Subjects # Conditions	Population and Study Characteristics	Teledermatology Characteristics	Outcomes Evaluated	Quality Rating
A. Store and forward systems studies (n=41)					
Warshaw 2009[5] United States, US armed service personnel/veterans Repeated Measure Funding: Department of Veterans Affairs Health Services R&D Service	542 542	Mean age (range): 66 years (23-94) Gender: female 4%, male 96% Race/ethnicity: white 97% Condition characteristics: Benign Neoplasm:267 Keratinocyte Carcinoma:84 Dysplastic Nevus: 155 Melanoma:36 Inclusion criteria: PSL Exclusion criteria: Skin tags, previously biopsied lesions Study duration (months): 3	Nikon Coolpix 4500, 3Gen Dermlite, Minolta X370 with Heine dermphot (TDSC) Photographer: Support staff Time between photograph and gold standard (days): 0	Diagnostic Accuracy: Yes Diagnostic Concordance: No Management Accuracy: Yes Management Concordance: No	Overall QUADAS score: 12/14 *Sources of bias identified by QUADAS* Selection: 1/2 Index test: 7/7 Reference test: 3/3 Data analysis: 1/2

**Teledermatology for Diagnosis and Management of Skin Conditions:
A Systematic Review of the Evidence**

Study Country Study design Funding	# Subjects # Conditions	Population and Study Characteristics	Teledermatology Character-istics	Outcomes Evaluated	Quality Rating
Warshaw 2009[6] United States, US armed service personnel/veterans Repeated Measure Funding: Department of Veterans Affairs Health Services R&D Service	728 728	Mean age (range): 71 years (21-94) Gender: female 2%, male 98% Race/ethnicity: white 99% Condition Characteristics: Keratinocyte Carcinoma - 385 Actinic Keratosis - 81 Benign Neoplasm - 258 Other - 4 Inclusion criteria: Non-pigmented neoplasms Exclusion criteria: Skin tags, previously biopsied lesions Study duration (months): 34	Nikon Coolpix 4500 3Gen Dermlite (TDSC) Photographer: Support staff Time between photograph and gold standard (days): 0	Diagnostic Accuracy: Yes Diagnostic Concordance: No Management Accuracy: Yes Management Concordance: No	Overall QUADAS score: 12/14 *Sources of bias identified by QUADAS* Selection: 1/2 Index test: 7/7 Reference test: 3/3 Data analysis: 1/2
Edison 2008[7] United States Repeated Measure Both SAF and LI Funding: Federal Office for the Advancement of Telehealth, Health Resources and Services Administration	110 110	Mean age (range): 42 (7-92) Gender: female 69%, male 31% Race/ethnicity: white 85%, black 12%, Asian 2%, Hispanic 1% Condition Characteristics (Only reported for 70): Actinic Keratosis - 10 Acneiform - 12 Benign Neoplasm - 19 Dysplastic nevus - 1 Infectious - 7 Eczematous - 8 Other – 13 Inclusion criteria: New pts on study days Exclusion criteria: NR Study duration (months): 18	Camera: NR Photographer: NR Time between photograph and gold standard (days): 0	Diagnostic Accuracy: No Diagnostic Concordance: Yes Management Accuracy: No Management Concordance: Yes	Overall QUADAS score: 11/14 *Sources of bias identified by QUADAS* Selection: 1/2 Index test: 7/7 Reference test: 3/3 Data analysis: 0/2

Study Country Study design Funding	# Subjects # Conditions	Population and Study Characteristics	Teledermatology Characteristics	Outcomes Evaluated	Quality Rating
Fabbrocini 2008[8] Italy Repeated Measure Funding: NR	NR 44	Age: NR Gender: NR Race/Ethnicity: NR Condition characteristics: Melanoma - 22 Benign Neoplasm - 15 Dysplastic nevi - 7 Inclusion criteria: Non-pigmented, absence of regular network, or diameter <5 mm Exclusion criteria: NR Study duration (months): NR	Nikon 4500 Coolpix, Wild M650 Steromicroscope Photographer: Dermatologist Time between photograph and gold standard (days): NR	Diagnostic Accuracy: Yes Diagnostic Concordance: No Management Accuracy: No Management Concordance: No	Overall QUADAS score: 8/14 *Sources of bias identified by QUADAS* Selection: 0/2 Index test: 7/7 Reference test: 1/3 Data analysis: 1/2
Di Stefani 2007[9] Italy Repeated Measure Funding: NR	18 465	Mean age (range): 28.4 years (10-55) Gender: female 39%, male 61% Race/ethnicity: NR Condition characteristics: PSL Inclusion criteria: ≥3 clinically atypical nevi on back Exclusion criteria: NR	Nikon 990 (macro), Videocap digital videodermoscopy Photographer: NR Time between photograph and gold standard (days): 0	Diagnostic Accuracy: No Diagnostic Concordance: No Management Accuracy: No Management Concordance: Yes	Overall QUADAS score: 11/14 *Sources of bias identified by QUADAS* Selection: 1/2 Index test: 7/7 Reference test: 3/3 Data analysis: 0/2

Teledermatology for Diagnosis and Management of Skin Conditions:
A Systematic Review of the Evidence

Study Country Study design Funding	# Subjects # Conditions	Population and Study Characteristics	Teledermatology Character-istics	Outcomes Evaluated	Quality Rating
Ferrandiz 2007[10] Spain Repeated Measure Funding: Instituto Carlos III	134 134	Mean age: 70.3 years Gender: female 39%, male 61% Race/ethnicity: NR Condition characteristics: Keratinocyte Carcinoma - 95 Actinic keratosis - 14 Melanoma - 1 Other - 3 Benign Neoplasm - 17 Inclusion criteria: Non-melanoma skin cancer or fast-growing vascular tumor Exclusion criteria: "Lesions expected to require major reconstruction", melanoma Study duration (months): 12	Nikon Coolpix 4300 Photographer: NR Time between photograph and gold standard (days): mean 26 days	Diagnostic Accuracy: Yes Diagnostic Concordance: No Management Accuracy: No Management Concordance: Yes	Overall QUADAS score: 9/14 *Sources of bias identified by QUADAS* Selection: 0/2 Index test: 6/7 Reference test: 3/3 Data analysis: 0/2
Moreno-Ramirez[11] 2007 Spain Repeated Measure Funding: Instituto Carlos III	882 890	Mean age: 41.5 years Gender: female 59%, male 41% Race/ethnicity: NR Condition characteristics: Benign Neoplasm - 548 Keratinocyte Carcinoma - 119 Actinic keratosis - 102 Melanoma - 18 Infectious - 9 Papulosquamous/Other - 15 Other Malignant Neoplasm - 3 Dysplastic nevus - 76 Inclusion criteria: Circumscribed lesions Exclusion criteria: NR Study duration (months): 15	Nikon Coolpix 4300 Photographer: NR Time between photograph and gold standard (days): <31	Diagnostic Accuracy: No Diagnostic Concordance: Yes Management Accuracy: No Management Concordance: No	Overall QUADAS score: 12/14 *Sources of bias identified by QUADAS* Selection: 1/2 Index test: 6/7 Reference test: 3/3 Data analysis: 2/2

Teledermatology for Diagnosis and Management of Skin Conditions: A Systematic Review of the Evidence

Study Country Study design Funding	# Subjects # Conditions	Population and Study Characteristics	Teledermatology Characteristics	Outcomes Evaluated	Quality Rating
Bowns 2006[12] United Kingdom Randomized controlled trial; Data extracted from TD arm Funding: National Health Service R&D grant	92 92	Mean age: intervention 43.6 years, Gender: female 63%, male 37% Race/ethnicity: NR Condition characteristics: Malignancy- 3 Benign Neoplasm –5 Infectious - 4 Eczematous – 11 Papulosquamous/Other - 62 Acneiform - 7 Inclusion criteria: ≥ 16 years old, had not seen dermatologist in last year Exclusion criteria: genital lesions Study duration (months): NR	Nikon Coolpix 900 Photographer: Primary care staff, often general practitioner Time between photograph and gold standard (days): mean 60	Diagnostic Accuracy: No Diagnostic Concordance: Yes Management Accuracy: No Management Concordance: Yes	Overall QUADAS score: 10/14 *Sources of bias identified by QUADAS* Selection: 2/2 Index test: 4/7 Reference test: 2/3 Data analysis: 2/2
Bowns 2006[13] United Kingdom Repeated Measure Funding: National Health Service R&D grant	256 256	Mean age: NR Gender: female 53%, male 47% Race/ethnicity: NR Condition characteristics: Keratinocyte Carcinoma – 54 Actinic keratosis–15 Dysplastic nevus-3 Melanoma-24 Benign neoplasm-159 Other-1 Inclusion criteria: Suspected skin cancer Exclusion criteria: NR Study duration (months): NR	Camera: NR Photographer: Medical Photography Department Time between photograph and gold standard (days): 0	Diagnostic Accuracy: No Diagnostic Concordance: Yes Management Accuracy: No Management Concordance: Yes	Overall QUADAS score: 11/14 *Sources of bias identified by QUADAS* Selection: 0/2 Index test: 6/7 Reference test: 3/3 Data analysis: 2/2

Teledermatology for Diagnosis and Management of Skin Conditions: A Systematic Review of the Evidence

Study Country Study design Funding	# Subjects # Conditions	Population and Study Characteristics	Teledermatology Character-istics	Outcomes Evaluated	Quality Rating
Moreno-Ramirez 2006[14] Spain Repeated Measure Funding: Instituto Carlos III	61 61	Mean age (range): 39 years (1-73) Gender: female 71%, male 29%, Race/ethnicity: NR Condition characteristics: Keratinocyte Carcinoma - 2 Benign Neoplasm - 54 Melanoma – 1 Dysplastic Nevus - 1 Inclusion criteria: PSL Exclusion criteria: Pts who did not show to CD Study duration (months): 2	Nikon Coolpix 4500 DermLite (TDSC) Photographer: General practitioner Time between photograph and gold standard (days): <30	Diagnostic Accuracy: Yes Diagnostic Concordance: No Management Accuracy: No Management Concordance: No	Overall QUADAS score: 11/14 *Sources of bias identified by QUADAS* Selection: 1/2 Index test: 6/7 Reference test: 3/3 Data analysis: 1/2
Oakley 2006[15] New Zealand Repeated Measure Funding: NR	73 109	Mean age (range): 59 years (16-93) Gender: female 64%, male 36% Race/ethnicity: NR Condition characteristics: Keratinocyte Carcinoma - 43 Actinic keratoses - 17 Melanoma – 8 Benign neoplasms - 37 Papulosquamous/Other - 4 Inclusion criteria: New pts with skin growth Exclusion criteria: Inflammatory dermatoses, infections, resolved lesions, poor quality images Study duration (months): NR	Nikon Coolpix 955 38 TD (6 were trainee dermatologists) Photographer: medical student Time between photograph and gold standard (days): 0	Diagnostic Accuracy: Yes Diagnostic Concordance: Yes Management Accuracy: No Management Concordance: Yes	Overall QUADAS score: 10/14 *Sources of bias identified by QUADAS* Selection: 0/2 Index test: 7/7 Reference test: 3/3 Data analysis: 0/2

Teledermatology for Diagnosis and Management of Skin Conditions:
A Systematic Review of the Evidence

Study Country Study design Funding	# Subjects # Conditions	Population and Study Characteristics	Teledermatology Character-istics	Outcomes Evaluated	Quality Rating
Baba 2005[17] Turkey Repeated Measure Both SAF and LI Funding: NR	228 242	Mean age (range): 35 years (2-82) Gender: female 63%, male 37% Race/ethnicity: NR Condition characteristics: Acneiform - 41 Infectious - 54 Pre-malignant/Malignant- 2 Eczematous - 46 Benign Neoplasms - 45 Papulosquamous/Other - 54 Inclusion criteria: New dermatology pts Exclusion criteria: None Study duration (months): 2.3	Canon Powershot S10 Two dermatologists with 3 to 5 years experience. Photographer: Nurse Time between photographing and gold standard test (days): NR	Diagnostic Accuracy: No Diagnostic Concordance: Yes Management Accuracy: No Management Concordance: No	Overall QUADAS score: 9/14 *Sources of bias identified by QUADAS* Selection: 1/2 Index test: 6/7 Reference test: 2/3 Data analysis: 0/2
Mahendran 2005[16] United Kingdom Repeated Measure Funding: NR	163 163	Age: NR Gender: NR Race/ethnicity: NR Condition characteristics: Benign Neoplasm - 81 Keratinocyte Carcinoma - 48 Actinic keratoses - 10 Melanoma - 5 Infectious - 3 Papulosquamous/Other - 10 Dysplastic nevus - 6 Inclusion criteria: Pts with suspected skin cancer, informed consent Exclusion criteria: Pts who did show to CD (number NR) Study duration (months): 18	Nikon Coolpix 950 2 different dermatologists and a 3rd year trainee dermatologist viewed all the cases as well Photographer: General practitioner Time between photograph and gold standard (days): <14	Diagnostic Accuracy: No Diagnostic Concordance: Yes Management Accuracy: No Management Concordance: Yes	Overall QUADAS score: 8/14 *Sources of bias identified by QUADAS* Selection: 0/2 Index test: 5/7 Reference test: 2/3 Data analysis: 1/2

Study Country Study design Funding	# Subjects # Conditions	Population and Study Characteristics	Teledermatology Character-istics	Outcomes Evaluated	Quality Rating
Moreno-Ramirez 2005[18] Spain Repeated Measure Funding: Grant from Instituto Carlos III	108 108	Mean age (range): 43 years (2 to 84) Gender: female 65%, male 35% Race/ethnicity: NR Condition characteristics (for 57 biopsied PSL): Keratinocyte Carcinoma - 23 Benign Neoplasm - 12 Dysplastic Nevi -16 Melanoma - 6 Inclusion criteria: changing, new, symptomatic or concerning pigmented lesions Exclusion criteria: NR Study duration (months): 3	Nikon Coolpix 4300 Photographer: General practitioner Time between photograph and gold standard (days): mean 8 days (range 5-14)	Diagnostic Accuracy: Yes Diagnostic Concordance: Yes Management Accuracy: No Management Concordance: No	Overall QUADAS score: 9/14 *Sources of bias identified by QUADAS* Selection: 0/2 Index test: 7/7 Reference test: 2/3 Data analysis: 0/2
Tucker 2005[19] United Kingdom Repeated Measure Funding: NR	75 84	Mean age: NR Gender: female 64%, male 36% Race/ethnicity: NR Condition characteristics: NR Inclusion criteria: NR Exclusion criteria: NR Study duration (months): 1	Fujifilm MX-1700 Photographer: dermatologists Time between photograph and gold standard (days): 0	Diagnostic Accuracy : No Diagnostic Concordance: Yes Management Accuracy: No Management Concordance: No	Overall QUADAS score: 10/14 *Sources of bias identified by QUADAS* Selection: 0/2 Index test: 7/7 Reference test: 3/3 Data analysis: 2/2

Teledermatology for Diagnosis and Management of Skin Conditions: A Systematic Review of the Evidence

Study Country Study design Funding	# Subjects # Conditions	Population and Study Characteristics	Teledermatology Character-istics	Outcomes Evaluated	Quality Rating
Ferrara 2004[21] Italy Repeated Measure Funding: NR	12 12	Median age (range): 41 years (14-71) Gender: female 17%, male 83% Race/ethnicity: NR Condition characteristics: PSL Benign Neoplasm - 5 Melanoma - 7 Inclusion criteria: NR Exclusion criteria: NR Study duration (months): NR	TDSC: Heine Dermaphot Molemax Videocap Photographer: NR Time between photograph and gold standard (days): NR	Diagnostic Accuracy: Yes Diagnostic Concordance: No Management Accuracy: No Management Concordance: No	Overall QUADAS score: 9/14 *Sources of bias identified by QUADAS* Selection: 0/2 Index test: 6/7 Reference test: 3/3 Data analysis: 0/2
Oztas 2004[20] Turkey Repeated Measure Funding: NR	125 125	Age: NR Gender: NR Race/ethnicity: NR Condition characteristics: Infectious - 50 Tumors (not further defined) -12 Eczematous - 10 Acneiform - 8 Papulosquamous/ Other - 39 Benign Neoplasm - 6 Inclusion criteria: NR Exclusion criteria: NR Study duration (months): NR	Canon Powershot 70 Photographer: NR Time between photograph and gold standard (days): NR	Diagnostic Accuracy: No Diagnostic Concordance: Yes Management Accuracy: No Management Concordance: No	Overall QUADAS score: 11/14 *Sources of bias identified by QUADAS* Selection: 1/2 Index test: 7/7 Reference test: 3/3 Data analysis: 0/2

Study Country Study design Funding	# Subjects # Conditions	Population and Study Characteristics	Teledermatology Character-istics	Outcomes Evaluated	Quality Rating
Piccolo 2004[22] Italy Repeated Measure Funding: NR	73 77	Mean age (range): 28 years (4-77) Gender: female 53%, male 47% Race/ethnicity: NR Condition characteristics: Acral PSL Benign - 71 Melanomas - 6 Inclusion criteria: Acral melanocytic lesions Exclusion criteria: NR Study duration (months): NR	TDSC: Molemax II, Heine Dermaphot Photographer: NR Time between photograph and gold standard (days): NR	Diagnostic Accuracy: Yes Diagnostic Concordance: No Management Accuracy: No Management Concordance: No	Overall QUADAS score: 9/14 *Sources of bias identified by QUADAS* Selection: 0/2 Index test: 7/7 Reference test: 2/3 Data analysis: 0/2
Shapiro 2004[23] United States Repeated Measure Funding: University of Pennsylvania Department of Dermatology	49 49	Mean age: NR Gender: female 46%, male 54% Race/ethnicity: NR Condition characteristics: Skin growths Inclusion criteria: Skin growth referred by general practitioner Exclusion criteria: Previous dermatology evaluation Study duration (months): NR	Olympus D-600L Photographer: General practitioner Time between photograph and gold standard (days): <16	Diagnostic Accuracy: No Diagnostic Concordance: No Management Accuracy: No Management Concordance: Yes	Overall QUADAS score: 11/14 *Sources of bias identified by QUADAS* Selection: 1/2 Index test: 7/7 Reference test: 3/3 Data analysis: 2/2

Study Country Study design Funding	# Subjects # Conditions	Population and Study Characteristics	Teledermatology Character-istics	Outcomes Evaluated	Quality Rating
Coras 2003[24] Germany Repeated Measure Funding: NR	NR 45	Age, gender, and race/ethnicity: NR Condition characteristics: PSL Benign Neoplasm - 24 Dysplastic Nevus - 5 Melanoma - 16 Inclusion criteria: NR Exclusion criteria: NR Study duration (months): 16	Dermogenius ultra Photographer: Clinic dermatoscopic examiner Time between photograph and gold standard (days): 0	Diagnostic Accuracy: Yes Diagnostic Concordance: No Management Accuracy: No Management Concordance: No	Overall QUADAS score: 11/14 *Sources of bias identified by QUADAS* Selection: 0/2 Index test: 7/7 Reference test: 3/3 Data analysis: 1/2
Du Moulin 2003[25] Netherlands Repeated Measure Funding: University Hospital Maastricht and Ministry of Economic Affairs	106 106	Mean age: 47 years Gender: NR Race/ethnicity: NR Condition characteristics: Malignant/Premalignant - 6 Benign Neoplasms - 12 Eczematous 28 Infectious- 15 Acneiform - 13 Papulosquamous/Other - 22 Inclusion criteria: Pts referred from general practitioner Exclusion criteria: Dermatologic referral clearly indicated Study Duration (months): 11	Ricoh 5000 Photographer: General practitioner Time between photograph and gold standard (days): 0	Diagnostic Accuracy: No Diagnostic Concordance: Yes Management Accuracy: No Management Concordance: No	Overall QUADAS score: 12/14 *Sources of bias identified by QUADAS* Selection: 2/2 Index test: 7/7 Reference test: 3/3 Data analysis: 0/2

83

Teledermatology for Diagnosis and Management of Skin Conditions: A Systematic Review of the Evidence

Study Country Study design Funding	# Subjects # Conditions	Population and Study Characteristics	Teledermatology Character-istics	Outcomes Evaluated	Quality Rating
Pak 2003 *(Part I[27] and Part II[26])* United States, 100% army veterans, or relatives Repeated Measure Funding: Walter Reed Army Medical Center	404 404	Mean age (range): 59 years (18-92) Gender: female 43%, male 57% Race/ethnicity: white 82%, black 13%, Asian/Hispanic 5% Condition characteristics: Infectious - 31 Premalignant/Malignant - 54 Acneiform - 28 Benign neoplasm - 115 Eczematous - 44 Papulosquamous/Other - 132 Inclusion criteria: Adult new pts Exclusion criteria: Medical emergencies Study duration (months): 4	Olympus D-600L Nikon Coolpix 900 Photographer: Nurse Time between photograph and gold standard (days): 0	Diagnostic Accuracy: Yes Diagnostic Concordance: Yes Management Accuracy: No Management Concordance: Yes	Overall QUADAS score: 10/14 *Sources of bias identified by QUADAS* Selection: 2/2 Index test: 6/7 Reference test: 2/3 Data analysis: 0/2
Rashid 2003[28] Pakistan Repeated Measure Funding: NR	33 33	Age, gender, and race/ethnicity: NR Condition characteristics: Keratinocyte Carcinoma - 1 Infectious - 9 Eczematous - 4 Benign Neoplasm - 3 Papulosquamous/Other - 16 Inclusion criteria: NR Exclusion criteria: Common conditions such as acne and melasma Study duration (months):NR	Kodak DC-210 Photographer: "Trainee doctor" Time between photograph and gold standard (days): NR	Diagnostic Accuracy: No Diagnostic Concordance: Yes Management Accuracy: No Management Concordance: No	Overall QUADAS score: 12/14 *Sources of bias identified by QUADAS* Selection: 1/2 Index test: 7/7 Reference test: 3/3 Data analysis: 1/2

Study Country Study design Funding	# Subjects # Conditions	Population and Study Characteristics	Teledermatology Character-istics	Outcomes Evaluated	Quality Rating
Oliveira 2002[29] Brazil Repeated Measure Funding: NR	92 NR	Age: NR Gender: NR Race/ethnicity: NR Condition characteristics: NR Inclusion criteria: NR Exclusion criteria: NR Study duration (months): NR	Kodak DC265 Photographer: nurse Time between photograph and gold standard (days): <7	Diagnostic Accuracy: No Diagnostic Concordance: Yes Management Accuracy: No Management Concordance: No	Overall QUADAS score: 9/14 *Sources of bias identified by QUADAS* Selection: 0/2 Index test: 6/7 Reference test: 2/3 Data analysis: 1/2
Jolliffe 2001[30] United Kingdom Repeated Measure Funding: National Health Service R&D grant	138 144	Age range: 15-94 years Gender: female 66%, male 34% Race/ethnicity: NR Condition characteristics: PSL Inclusion criteria: PSL Exclusion criteria: NR Study duration (months): NR	Sanyo HiFi video Photographer: Dermatologist Time between photograph and gold standard (days): NR	Diagnostic Accuracy: Yes Diagnostic Concordance: No Management Accuracy: No Management Concordance: No	Overall QUADAS score: 11/14 *Sources of bias identified by QUADAS* Selection: 0/2 Index test: 7/7 Reference test: 3/3 Data analysis: 1/2

Study Country Study design Funding	# Subjects # Conditions	Population and Study Characteristics	Teledermatology Character-istics	Outcomes Evaluated	Quality Rating
Jolliffe 2001[31] United Kingdom Repeated Measure Funding: National Health Service Executive London R&D grant	611 819	Age range: 8 to 94 years Gender: female 76%, male 24% Race/ethnicity: NR Condition characteristics: PSL Benign Neoplasm - 635 Keratinocyte Carcinoma - 20 Dysplastic Nevi - 112 Actinic keratoses - 13 Melanoma - 9 Infectious - 10 Acneiform - 5 Rash/Other - 13 Eczematous - 2 Inclusion criteria: PSL Exclusion criteria: Genital lesions, mental impairment, fear of technical equipment Study duration (months): NR	Sanyo HiFi video Photographer: Dermatologist Time between photograph and gold standard (days): NR	Diagnostic Accuracy: No Diagnostic Concordance: No Management Accuracy: No Management Concordance: Yes	Overall QUADAS score: 9/14 *Sources of bias identified by QUADAS* Selection: 0/2 Index test: 6/7 Reference test: 2/3 Data analysis: 1/2

Study Country Study design Funding	# Subjects # Conditions	Population and Study Characteristics	Teledermatology Character-istics	Outcomes Evaluated	Quality Rating
Lim 2001[32] Australia Repeated Measure Funding: Australian Dermatology Research and Education Foundation	23 27	Age: NR Gender: NR Race/ethnicity: NR Condition Characteristics: Eczematous - 18 Benign Neoplasm - 9 Infectious - 12 Keratinocyte Carcinoma - 3 Acneiform - 6 Paulosquamous/Other - 5 Inclusion criteria: new skin condition Exclusion criteria: wart or acne Study duration (months): 3	Kodak DC265 Photographer: Dermatologist Time between photograph and gold standard (days): ≤7	Diagnostic Accuracy: No Diagnostic Concordance: Yes Management Accuracy: No Management Concordance: No	Overall QUADAS score: 10/14 *Sources of bias identified by QUADAS* Selection: 1/2 Index test: 7/7 Reference test: 1/3 Data analysis: 0/2
Taylor 2001[33] United Kingdom Repeated Measure Funding: NR	188 NR	Age: NR Gender: NR Race/ethnicity: "42% of the conditions from pigmented pts" Condition characteristics (most common diagnoses in 127): Eczematous - 21 Keratinocyte carcinoma - 9 Papulosquamous/Other - 15 Benign Neoplasm - 69 Acneiform - 8 Infectious - 5 Inclusion criteria: New dermatology pts Exclusion criteria: NR Study duration (months): 3	NR Photographer: Nurse Time between photograph and gold standard test: NR	Diagnostic Accuracy: No Diagnostic Concordance: Yes Management Accuracy: No Management Concordance: No	Overall QUADAS score: 13/14 *Sources of bias identified by QUADAS* Selection: 1/2 Index test: 7/7 Reference test: 3/3 Data analysis: 2/2

Study Country Study design Funding	# Subjects # Conditions	Population and Study Characteristics	Teledermatology Character-istics	Outcomes Evaluated	Quality Rating
Barnard 2000[34] United States Repeated Measure Funding: NR	50 "cases"	Age: NR Gender: NR Race/ethnicity: NR Condition characteristics: 8 skin cancer cases Inclusion criteria: NR Exclusion criteria: NR Study duration (months): NR	Nikon Fujix DS505, Nikon SLR Photographer: NR Time between photograph and gold standard (days): NR	Diagnostic Accuracy: Yes Diagnostic Concordance: Yes Management Accuracy: No Management Concordance: No	Overall QUADAS score: 10/14 *Sources of bias identified by QUADAS* Selection: 0/2 Index test: 7/7 Reference test: 3/3 Data analysis: 0/2
Braun 2000[35] Switzerland Repeated Measure Funding: NR	51 55	Age: NR Gender: NR Race/ethnicity: NR Condition characteristics: PSL Benign Neoplasm - 37 Dysplastic Nevus - 3 Melanoma - 9 Keratinocyte Carcinoma - 4 Other -2 Inclusion criteria: NR Exclusion criteria: NR Study duration (months): 6	TDSC: Mitsubishi CCD Photographer: 6 dermatologists Time between photograph and gold standard (days): NR	Diagnostic Accuracy: Yes Diagnostic Concordance: No Management Accuracy: No Management Concordance: No	Overall QUADAS score: 10/14 *Sources of bias identified by QUADAS* Selection: 0/2 Index test: 7/7 Reference test: 2/3 Data analysis: 1/2

Teledermatology for Diagnosis and Management of Skin Conditions:
A Systematic Review of the Evidence

Study Country Study design Funding	# Subjects # Conditions	Population and Study Characteristics	Teledermatology Character-istics	Outcomes Evaluated	Quality Rating
High 2000[36] United States Repeated Measure Funding: Mayo Clinic and Foundation, Minnesota Academy of Family Physicians	92 106	Mean age (range): 39.7 years (10 months - 81 years) Gender: female 48%, male 52% Race/ethnicity: NR Condition characteristics: Benign Neoplasm - 35 Keratinocyte Carcinoma - 6 Actinic keratoses -2 Melanoma - 1 Infectious - 12 Acneiform - 8 Papulosquamous/Other - 25 Eczematous - 17 Inclusion criteria: NR Exclusion criteria: None Study duration (months): 1.5	Sony DCS-F1 Photographer: Medical student Time between photograph and gold standard (days): NR	Diagnostic Accuracy: No Diagnostic Concordance: Yes Management Accuracy: No Management Concordance: No	Overall QUADAS score: 11/14 *Sources of bias identified by QUADAS* Selection: 1/2 Index test: 7/7 Reference test: 3/3 Data analysis: 0/2
Piccolo 2000[37] Italy Repeated Measure Funding: Osterreichische Krebshilfe Steiermark, Graz, Austria	40 43	Mean age (range): 39.5 years (3-91) Gender: female 47.5%, male 52.5% Race/ethnicity: NR Condition characteristics: PSL Keratinocyte carcinoma - 3 Melanoma - 11 Benign Neoplasm - 29 Inclusion criteria: NR Exclusion criteria: NR Study duration (months): 3	TDSC: video camera and stereomicroscope Photographer: NR Time between photograph and gold standard (days): NR	Diagnostic Accuracy: Yes Diagnostic Concordance: No Management Accuracy: No Management Concordance: No	Overall QUADAS score: 10/14 *Sources of bias identified by QUADAS* Selection: 0/2 Index test: 7/7 Reference test: 3/3 Data analysis: 0/2

Teledermatology for Diagnosis and Management of Skin Conditions: A Systematic Review of the Evidence

Study Country Study design Funding	# Subjects # Conditions	Population and Study Characteristics	Teledermatology Character-istics	Outcomes Evaluated	Quality Rating
Krupinski 1999[38] United States Repeated Measure Funding: USDA Rural Utilities Service , US Dept. of Commerce, Health and Human Services	308 308	Age, gender, and race/ethnicity: NR Condition characteristics: Melanoma - 4 Actinic keratoses - 20 Keratinocyte Carcinoma - 49 Dysplastic nevus - 16 Benign Neoplasm - 106 Infection - 20 Eczematous - 36 Papulosquamous/Other - 57 Inclusion criteria: NR Exclusion criteria: NR Study duration (months): NR	Canon Powershot 600 Photographer: Medical students Time between photograph and gold standard (days): NR	Diagnostic Accuracy: Yes Diagnostic Concordance: Yes Management Accuracy: No Management Concordance: No	Overall QUADAS score: 10/14 *Sources of bias identified by QUADAS* Selection: 1/2 Index test: 7/7 Reference test: 2/3 Data analysis: 0/2
Lewis 1999[39] United Kingdom Repeated Measure Funding: NR	56 cases	Age: NR Gender: NR Race/ethnicity: NR Condition characteristics: NR Inclusion criteria: NR Exclusion criteria: NR Study duration (months): 7	Kodak DC40 Photographer: NR Time between photograph and gold standard (days): 0	Diagnostic Accuracy: No Diagnostic Concordance: Yes Management Accuracy: No Management Concordance: No	Overall QUADAS score: 8/14 *Sources of bias identified by QUADAS* Selection: 0/2 Index test: 5/7 Reference test: 3/3 Data analysis: 0/2

Study Country Study design Funding	# Subjects # Conditions	Population and Study Characteristics	Teledermatology Character-istics	Outcomes Evaluated	Quality Rating
Piccolo 1999[40] Italy Repeated Measure Funding: NR	66 66	Mean age (range): 41.2 years (8-82) Gender: female 52%, male 48% Race/ethnicity: NR Condition characteristics: PSL Melanocytic- 57 Nonmelanocytic-9 Inclusion criteria: NR Exclusion criteria: NR Study duration (months): 0.75	TDSC: video camera and stereomicroscope Photographer: NR Time between photograph and gold standard (days): NR	Diagnostic Accuracy: Yes Diagnostic Concordance: Yes Management Accuracy: No Management Concordance: No	Overall QUADAS score: 10/14 *Sources of bias identified by QUADAS* Selection: 0/2 Index test: 7/7 Reference test: 3/3 Data analysis: 0/2
Tait 1999[41] Australia Repeated Measure Funding: NR	30 NR	Age: NR Gender: NR Race/ethnicity: NR Condition characteristics: NR Inclusion criteria: Visible skin lesion Exclusion criteria: NR Study duration (months): NR	Ricoh RDC 300 Photographer: NR Time between photograph and gold standard (days): 0	Diagnostic Accuracy: No Diagnostic Concordance: Yes Management Accuracy: No Management Concordance: No	Overall QUADAS score: 10/14 *Sources of bias identified by QUADAS* Selection: 2/2 Index test: 6/7 Reference test: 2/3 Data analysis: 0/2
Whited 1999[42] United States, US armed service personnel/veterans Repeated Measure Funding: Veterans Affairs Health Service R&D	129 168	Mean age (range): 61 years (22 to 82) Gender: female 2%, male 98% Race/ethnicity: white 80%, black 20% Condition characteristics: NR Inclusion criteria: Diagnostic uncertainty Exclusion criteria: Previous dermatology evaluation Study duration (months): NR	Fujix DS-515 Photographer: Research assistant Time between photograph and gold standard (days): 0	Diagnostic Accuracy: Yes Diagnostic Concordance: Yes Management Accuracy: No Management Concordance: Yes	Overall QUADAS score: 10/14 *Sources of bias identified by QUADAS* Selection: 0/2 Index test: 7/7 Reference test: 3/3 Data analysis: 0/2

Study Country Study design Funding	# Subjects # Conditions	Population and Study Characteristics	Teledermatology Character- istics	Outcomes Evaluated	Quality Rating
Whited 1998[43] United States, VA pts Repeated Measure Funding: NR	12 13	Age: NR Gender: NR Race/ethnicity: NR Condition Characteristics: Benign neoplasm - 2 Keratinocyte carcinoma - 7 Actinic keratoses – 1 Other – 1 No biopsy - 1 Inclusion criteria: Suspected skin cancer Exclusion criteria: NR Study duration (months): NR	Fujix DS-515 digital camera, 1280x1000 pixels Photographer: NR Time between photograph and gold standard test (days): 0	Diagnostic Accuracy: Yes Diagnostic Concordance: Yes Management Accuracy: No Management Concordance: Yes	Overall QUADAS score: 10/14 *Sources of bias identified by QUADAS* Selection: 0/2 Index test: 7/7 Reference test: 3/3 Data analysis: 0/2
Kvedar 1997[44] United States Repeated Measure Funding: Massachusetts General Hospital Dermatology Service	116 123	Mean age (range): 40 years (18-84) Gender: NR Race/ethnicity: NR Condition characteristics: NR Inclusion criteria: NR Exclusion criteria: Acne or warts cases Study duration (months): 2	Kodak DCS 420 Photographer: Non- dermatologists Time between photograph and gold standard (days): 0	Diagnostic Accuracy: No Diagnostic Concordance: Yes Management Accuracy: No Management Concordance: No	Overall QUADAS score: 13/14 *Sources of bias identified by QUADAS* Selection: 2/2 Index test: 7/7 Reference test: 3/3 Data analysis: 1/2

Study Country Study design Funding	# Subjects # Conditions	Population and Study Characteristics	Teledermatology Charac-teristics	Outcomes Evaluated	Quality Rating
Lyon 1997[45] United Kingdom Repeated Measure Funding: NR	100 100	Age: NR Gender: NR Race/ethnicity: NR Condition characteristics: Eczematous - 12 Acneiform - 3 Infectious - 5 Other - 20 Benign Neoplasm - 41 Keratinocyte Carcinoma - 19 Actinic keratoses - 5 Inclusion criteria: Dermatology referral Exclusion criteria: NR Study duration (months): NR	DC-40 Kodak Photographer: Dermatology resident Time between photograph and gold standard (days): NR	Diagnostic Accuracy: No Diagnostic Concordance: Yes Management Accuracy: No Management Concordance: Yes	Overall QUADAS score: 8/14 *Sources of bias identified by QUADAS* Selection: 1/2 Index test: 4/7 Reference test: 3/3 Data analysis: 0/2
Zelickson 1997[46] United States Repeated Measure Funding: NR	29 30	Age: NR Gender: NR Race/ethnicity: NR Condition characteristics: Rash-18 Lesion-12 Inclusion criteria: Nursing home resident with a skin condition Exclusion criteria: NR Study duration (months): NR	Sony CCD-TR400 video Photographer: Nurse Time between photograph and gold standard (days): <2	Diagnostic Accuracy: No Diagnostic Concordance: Yes Management Accuracy: No Management Concordance: Yes	Overall QUADAS score: 11/14 *Sources of bias identified by QUADAS* Selection: 1/2 Index test: 7/7 Reference test: 3/3 Data analysis: 0/2

| Study
Country
Study design
Funding | #
Subjects
Conditions | Population and Study Characteristics | Teledermatology Charac-teristics | Outcomes Evaluated | Quality Rating |
|---|---|---|---|---|---|
| **B. Live interactive studies (n=10)** | | | | | |
| Edison 2008[7]

United States

Repeated Measure
Both SAF and LI

Funding: Federal
Office for the
Advancement
of Telehealth,
Health Resources
and Services
Administration | 110

110 | Mean age (range): 42 (7-92)
Gender: female 69%, male 31%
Race/ethnicity: white 85%, black 12%, Asian 2%, Hispanic 1%

Condition Characteristics for 70:
Actinic Keratosis - 10
Acneiform - 12
Benign Neoplasm - 19
Dysplastic nevus - 1
Infectious - 7
Eczematous - 8
Other – 13

Inclusion criteria: New pts on study days
Exclusion criteria: NR

Study duration (months): 18 | Camera: NR

Photographer: NR

Time between photograph and gold standard (days): 0 | Diagnostic Accuracy: No

Diagnostic Concordance: Yes

Management Accuracy: No

Management Concordance: Yes | Overall QUADAS score: 12/14
Sources of bias identified by QUADAS
Selection: 1/2
Index test: 7/7
Reference test: 3/3
Data analysis: 1/2 |

Study Country Study design Funding	# Subjects # Conditions	Population and Study Characteristics	Teledermatology Characteristics	Outcomes Evaluated	Quality Rating
Baba 2005[17] Turkey Repeated Measure SAF +LI Funding: NR	228 242	Mean age (range): 35 years (2-82) Gender: female 63%, male 37% Race/ethnicity: NR Condition characteristics: Acneiform - 41 Infectious - 54 Pre-malignant/Malignant- 2 Eczematous - 46 Benign Neoplasms - 45 Papulosquamous/Other - 54 Inclusion criteria: None Exclusion criteria: None Study duration (months): 2.3	Mustek camera Photographer: Nurse Time between photograph and gold standard (days): NR	Diagnostic Accuracy: No Diagnostic Concordance: Yes Management Accuracy: No Management Concordance: No	Overall QUADAS score: 11/14 *Sources of bias identified by QUADAS* Selection: 1/2 Index test: 7/7 Reference test: 3/3 Data analysis: 0/2
Nordal 2001[47] Norway Repeated Measure Funding:	112 112	Mean age (range): 40 years (17-82) Gender: female 51%, male 49% Race/ethnicity: NR Condition characteristics: Eczematous - 7 Acneiform - 1 Papulosquamous/Other - 6 Benign neoplasm - 1 Inclusion criteria: New dermatologic conditions Exclusion criteria: Surgical treatment, emergency cases and most nevi Study duration (months): NR	Sony CCD DXC 930P video Photographer: General practitioner Time between photograph and gold standard (days): NR	Diagnostic Accuracy: No Diagnostic Concordance: Yes Management Accuracy: No Management Concordance: No	Overall QUADAS score: 13/14 *Sources of bias identified by QUADAS* Selection: 2/2 Index test: 6/7 Reference test: 3/3 Data analysis: 2/2

Teledermatology for Diagnosis and Management of Skin Conditions:
A Systematic Review of the Evidence

Study Country Study design Funding	# Subjects # Conditions	Population and Study Characteristics	Teledermatology Characteristics	Outcomes Evaluated	Quality Rating
Gilmour 1998[48] United Kingdom Repeated Measure Funding: National Health Service	126 155	Age range: 3 month -83 years Gender: female 51%, male 49% Race/ethnicity: NR Condition characteristics: Eczematous - 55 Papulosquamous/Other - 37 Infection - 23 Acneiform - 12 Tumor - 20 Inclusion criteria: NR Exclusion criteria: NR Study duration (months): 12	Camera NR Photographer: General practitioner or trained assistant Time between photograph and gold standard (days): 0	Diagnostic Accuracy: No Diagnostic Concordance: Yes Management Accuracy: No Management Concordance: Yes	Overall QUADAS score: 9/14 *Sources of bias identified by QUADAS* Selection: 1/2 Index test: 6/7 Reference test: 2/3 Data analysis: 0/2
Lesher 1998[49] United States Repeated Measure Funding: Telemedicine Center of Medical College of Georgia	60 68	Age: ≥ 18 years of age Gender: NR Race/ethnicity: NR Condition characteristics: Eczematous -17 Benign Neoplasm -12 Keratinocyte Carcinoma - 3 Actinic keratosis - 6 Infectious - 4 Acneiform - 11 Papulosquamous/Other -15 Inclusion criteria: Adults with skin condition Exclusion criteria: NR Study duration (months): NR	VC TK-1280U, Panasonic WV-E550 Photographer: NR Time between photograph and gold standard (days): 0	Diagnostic Accuracy: No Diagnostic Concordance: Yes Management Accuracy: No Management Concordance: No	Overall QUADAS score: 11/14 *Sources of bias identified by QUADAS* Selection: 1/2 Index test: 7/7 Reference test: 3/3 Data analysis: 0/2

Study Country Study design Funding	# Subjects # Conditions	Population and Study Characteristics	Teledermatology Characteristics	Outcomes Evaluated	Quality Rating
Loane, 1998[50] United Kingdom Repeated Measure Funding: National Health Service	351 427	Mean age (range): 41 years (5 months-89 years) Gender: female 55%, male 45% Race/ethnicity: NR Condition characteristics (preliminary results): Tumor - 78 Eczema - 54 Infection - 28 Benign Neoplasm - 21 Acneiform - 13 Papulosquamous/Other - 42 Inclusion criteria: Dermatology referral Exclusion criteria: NR Study duration (months): 18	VC7000 video, KY-F55B JVC video Photographer: General practitioner Time between photograph and gold standard (days): 0	Diagnostic Accuracy: No Diagnostic Concordance: Yes Management Accuracy: No Management Concordance: Yes	Overall QUADAS score: 9/14 *Sources of bias identified by QUADAS* Selection: 1/2 Index test: 6/7 Reference test: 2/3 Data analysis: 0/2
Lowitt 1998[51] United States, US armed service personnel/veterans Repeated Measure Funding: Baltimore Research and Education Foundation	102 130	Median age (range): 65 (range 23 to 85) Gender: male 95%, female 5% Race/ethnicity: white 60%, black 40% Condition characteristics: Acneiform - 17 Eczematous - 33 Infectious - 9 Papulosquamous/Other -17 Benign Neoplasm - 36 Premalignant Tumor - 16 Malignant Neoplasm - 6 Inclusion criteria: consecutive dermatology outpts Exclusion criteria: Pts transported by stretcher Study duration (months): 2	3-CCS JVC video Photographer: Nurse escort Time between photograph and gold standard (days): 0	Diagnostic Accuracy: Yes Diagnostic Concordance: Yes Management Accuracy: No Management Concordance: No	Overall QUADAS score: 12/14 *Sources of bias identified by QUADAS* Selection: 2/2 Index test: 7/7 Reference test: 3/3 Data analysis: 0/2

**Teledermatology for Diagnosis and Management of Skin Conditions:
A Systematic Review of the Evidence**

Study Country Study design Funding	# Subjects # Conditions	Population and Study Characteristics	Teledermatology Charac- teristics	Outcomes Evaluated	Quality Rating
Phillips 1998[52] United States Repeated Measure Funding: NR	51 107	Mean age: 47 Gender: female 84%, male 16% Race/ethnicity: NR Condition characteristics: Benign Neoplasm - 81 Keratinocyte Carcicnoma - 5 Melanoma - 1 Premalignant - 14 Dysplastic Nevi - 5 Inclusion criteria: NR Exclusion criteria: NR Study duration (months): NR	Panasonic video, Canon video Photographer: Dermatologist Time between photograph and gold standard (days): NR	Diagnostic Accuracy: No Diagnostic Concordance: Yes Management Accuracy: No Management Concordance: Yes	Overall QUADAS score: 10/14 *Sources of bias identified by QUADAS* Selection: 0/2 Index test: 7/7 Reference test: 3/3 Data analysis: 0/2
Oakley 1997[53] New Zealand Repeated Measure Funding: Waikato Information Ser- vices Department of Health	104 135	Age range: 2-86 years, Gender: female 60%, male 40% Race/ethnicity: NR Condition characteristics: Eczematous - 17 Benign Neoplasm - 24 Malignant Neoplasm - 25 Actinic Keratosis - 15 Infectious - 7 Acneiform - 13 Melanoma - 4 Papulosquamous/Other –30 Inclusion criteria: New dermatology pts Exclusion criteria: NR Study duration (months): NR	Canon VC-C1 video, Vtel system Photographer: Dermatologist Time between photograph and gold standard (days): 0	Diagnostic Accuracy: No Diagnostic Concordance: Yes Management Accuracy: No Management Concordance: No	Overall QUADAS score: 9/14 *Sources of bias identified by QUADAS* Selection: 1/2 Index test: 6/7 Reference test: 2/3 Data analysis: 0/2

Study Country Study design Funding	# Subjects # Conditions	Population and Study Characteristics	Teledermatology Charac-teristics	Outcomes Evaluated	Quality Rating
Phillips 1997[54] United States Repeated Measure Funding: NR	60 79	Mean age (range): 37 years (1-68) Gender: female, 60%, male 40% Race/ethnicity: white 73%, black 25% Condition characteristics: Eczematous - 14 NMSC - 4 Actinic keratosis - 5 Acneiform - 9 Infection - 8 Melanoma - 1 Benign Neoplasm - 26 Papulosquamous/Other -12 Inclusion criteria: Referral Exclusion criteria: NR Study duration (months): NR	Picture-Tel System 4000 video, Elmo model MN401X dc Photographer: trained nurse Time between photograph and gold standard (days): NR	Diagnostic Accuracy: No Diagnostic Concordance: Yes Management Accuracy: No Management Concordance: No	Overall QUADAS score: 10/14 *Sources of bias identified by QUADAS* Selection: 0/2 Index test: 7/7 Reference test: 3/3 Data analysis: 0/2